D0122163

PMSL

PMSL

Or How I Literally Pissed Myself Laughing and Survived the Last Taboo to Tell the Tale

LUCE BRETT

GREEN TREE
LONDON · OXFORD · NEW YORK · NEW DELHI · SYDNEY

GREEN TREE
Bloomsbury Publishing Plc
50 Bedford Square London WC1B 3DP UK

BLOOMSBURY, GREEN TREE and the Green Tree logo are trademarks of
Bloomsbury Publishing Plc

First published in Great Britain 2020

A catalogue record for this book is available from the British Library

Library of Congress Cataloguing-in-Publication data has been applied for

ISBN: HB: 978-1-4729-7748-9; eBook: 978-1-4729-7747-2

2 4 6 8 10 9 7 5 3 1

Typeset in Fournier by Deanta Global Publishing Services, Chennai, India
Printed and bound in Great Britain by CPI Group (UK) Ltd., Croydon, CR0 4YY

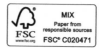

To find out more about our authors and books visit www.bloomsbury.com
and sign up for our newsletters

For leaky people everywhere

Hang on …

'stigma'
NOUN

'(1) A mark of disgrace associated with a particular circumstance, quality, or person.'

Oxford Living Dictionaries

…

'Bladder weakness alone affects 1 in 3 people and is more common than hay fever.'

World Federation of Incontinence Patients

Contents

CONTENTS

Introduction by Elaine Miller
Physiotherapist, Comedian,
Fellow of Chartered Society of Physiotherapists

There are some questions which are unwelcome, like 'Did you used to be a pretty lady, Mummy?' or, 'How did you get invited?' but, 'Do you wet yourself?' has to be one of the most awkward. Such is the silence which surrounds incontinence it's a question that's rarely asked – and one most of us would answer with a tinkly laugh and a firm lie. I get to ask that question to people every day because I'm a pelvic health physiotherapist.

The stats for incontinence are really depressing reading – one in three women wet themselves, and about one in 10 have problems controlling their bowels; isn't that shocking? Look at your office, your bus, your sports class, your home – if there are three females there, then one is probably thinking about her bladder and bowel most of the time. Leaking affects women of all ages, race and class – women who have not had kids, ones who had a birth injury, sporty women, sedentary women – basically, the science says that if you are female you are at risk of incontinence. I think we need to talk about this more, which is why I was so delighted when Luce said she was writing this book.

I also think the figures are too low. Embarrassment silences us. It's an unusual person who, when asked, 'Excuse me, do you wet yourself?' says, 'Yes, I do.'

I'm hard to embarrass. Pee, poo and sexual function are my favourite topics of conversation. Your pelvic floor is like a reliable legal system – you really don't notice it's there day to day, but, without it, life is chaos. Most of my days in clinic are spent elbow deep in leaky ladies, trying to jigsaw their continence back together. I love my job – living with incontinence takes a huge amount of preplanning and organising and worst-case-scenario prep, and I like seeing women restored to being able to leave the house without a giant bag containing a couple of changes of clothes and a plan B in it. The stories I hear in clinic of when the worst-case-scenario happened are always upsetting: incontinence can ruin lives.

One of my frustrations is that it often takes years for a woman to seek help, which is a shame because physio works for the majority of us. I wondered whether humour might help break down the taboos and embarrassment which prevent help-seeking, so I did the obvious thing – combined my hobby of stand-up comedy with work, and wrote an Edinburgh Fringe show about pelvic floors. I knew that comedy could be an effective health promotion tool and that the trick was making sure that it is the problem, not the person with the problem, who is the butt of the joke.

The parenting website, Mumsnet, had a motherload of stories about birth injuries, prolapse, and piles. There were pages and pages of women talking honestly about their experiences; only able to be brutally honest because they were anonymous.

That's where I first had the pleasure of Luce Brett's writing, discovering her blog about urodynamic testing (*see* Chapter 14). It was a comprehensive, funny, sweary, and raw look at a bread-and-butter investigation in clinic – and it was brilliant. Her account of the investigation had me totally hooked. I'd never had the investigation myself and she made me laugh out loud with the ridiculousness of how badly clinicians complicate things. She was also prepared to use some choice language to get to the heart of her anger and anxiety, to help me as a reader understand exactly how she felt, even when those feelings were really difficult. I wanted to find this brilliant woman and convince her to be my friend. So I did, and we have subjected our pelvic floors to many challenges with laughter and wine.

There are not many people who can advocate for themselves, and therefore for us all, in the way Luce has here. She is a patient expert, 'empowered with the skills, confidence and knowledge needed to play an active role in making informed decisions about their own health care and management of their chronic condition'. Health services need patient experts to show us what could be done better (like the, 'Where do I put my knickers when I take them off for an examination/procedure?' issue) and to remind us to keep our compassion burning when everyone is time-short and resource-poor (surely, a 'Put your knickers here' receptacle is an obvious clinic necessity?).

This book should be compulsory reading for all healthcare professionals. It gently reminds us that behind the symptom and the system there is a whole person. There are some shining examples of good, kind care in here. As you'll see, we should all aim to #BeMoreCarol.

Luce has somehow managed to put the fun into bladder dysfunction. She has a rare gift of being able to describe the indignity of living with incontinence with humour that doesn't diminish the challenges she faces, or her outrage that, statistically speaking, many women face an unnecessarily leaky, traumatised, depressed and inactive future.

Talking is kryptonite to taboos, and I am confident that this book will get us talking about these important and intimate problems – and redress the isolation and shame that prevents people from seeking help.

If you have a bladder or a bowel you should read this book.

E.M.
January, 2020

3

Prologue: The Beginning: How did I get here?

September 2007, outbuilding, large teaching hospital, London

The first time I meet a women's health physiotherapist, I'm frightened. I am also stressed, confused and late. I have so many fears and questions but mostly I'm preoccupied with language. How, I'm thinking, do I refer to my damaged bits? Is a physio chattier than a doctor? If I go biological I might muddle up my labia and my vulva and look like a fool, especially as I'm not altogether sure what's been stitched where, where the scars begin and I end. And if I don't speak properly, what do I do instead? Sink down into the vocabulary of *Viz*? Let my fear take over and debase us both by being crude and vulgar?

I'm still pondering this when I'm called in by a young Australian woman, who guides me down a long corridor past offices, gyms and rooms full of crutches. This is a space for people with proper injuries. Her room has no crutches. It has a sink, a bed, a desk and chairs, and an anatomy poster blu-tacked to the wall. The poster has a side-on illustration of a baby emerging from a birth canal. Gliding out of the opening, no blood, no fuss.

She asks about my recent experience giving birth and I recite the highlights, like a poem learned for school; I am *practised* at the chronology by now. I can drill down to the key information that medical types want: first baby, first pregnancy, to term, live birth, 'spontaneous vaginal delivery', no previous incontinence. I sound robotic, but I can't bear to add emotion.

Her twenty-something skin is luminous but she's an old hand at this, I think. She's nodding, sighing, raising eyebrows – all on cue. I can't focus too closely though, in case she's nice, so I tell my birth story to a dusty plastic pelvis model that she has on her shelf.

She asks for a list of things that make me leak – my first incontinence homework. I begin: 'Walking, running, stretching, coughing, sneezing, lifting up a baby, farting, shouting, crying, standing up, long strides, buses, exercise, stairs …'

I look up. She's just staring. I had her at 'farting'.

It's so unthinkingly intimate that it's only when I'm lying on the bed, bottom-half naked on the paper sheeting, about to be examined with my knees bent like a crazy pretzel, that I realise I don't know her name.

It seems the wrong moment to ask.

'A little bit cold now…' she says, and launches in. Her hand's a Girl Guide's salute and cold and slippy from the gloves and lube. She has 'exercises' she wants me to do. Lifts and squeezes. Long and short, where I am supposed to clench onto her fingers. I can feel her knuckles but I have to concentrate hard to squeeze any of it, to get a grip, especially because I'm also trying to follow her other instruction: 'Don't be embarrassed, Luce.'

I apologise. I don't want to do it wrong, though the truth is I can't really believe this is happening to me. The baby books didn't say anything about the etiquette for small talk while being fingered.

'Try to relax,' she says, as I try to ignore the fact that she's just checked my 'anal wink' and I flinched. I shouldn't find the word 'anal' impossibly grim – I'm a grown-up. But I'm at crunch point. The last few weeks have been a heady brew of shock, exhaustion, old wives' tales and humiliation and I just want a reset button. For my life to reboot and start again at the moment I became a mother. Or maybe just afterwards, when I had had a wash. Instead, I have this.

I lock onto the baby on the poster, his eyes closed, folded like a frog, he's edging out of his mother bloodlessly. I feel on the edge. But I am by nature compliant and enthusiastic.

'*In for a penny,*' I think, squeezing and holding and squeezing and holding as she counts it out. I can get through this. I am an adult woman and she's not the first person to check my mangled minge for damage. And maybe, unlike the others, this woman, with her sporty polo shirt, can at least offer me some practical help. Especially with the clenching and clunging.

My mind drifts to my baby boy in the waiting room with my friend. He's uncurling daily, opening up like a cabbage. He sleeps with his arms outstretched, a pudgy Jesus with curious black eyes. My tits twang at the thought of him. But the moment is ruined when the light from the window streams into my eyes. Windows remind me of the labour ward. They make me feel scared and weird.

I close my eyes again and keep it together with my legs apart. The physio is asking for me to clamp right down now. She says, 'Hold, hold, hold.'

I can't really feel what I'm doing, but I'm a fast learner, and I make up for technique with willpower and enthusiasm. Also, fear. She STILL has her hand inside me so I don't want to piss her off. I clamp and clench and pull and hold. Quite the performance. I want to be a star patient, almost as much as I want to get back to being me again.

And then it's over.

'Just pop your clothes on and we can have a chat,' she says, snapping off her gloves.

We make small talk as I dress, wiping myself clean-ish with paper towels. There was nowhere to put my clothes, so they were scrunched up on a chair, rolled up into a ball as I was scared she'd see the pad in my knickers. Our words chime into the empty air as she asks what plans I have for the rest of the day. I'll probably spend the afternoon lying with my son under the dining room table. He seems to prefer staring at corners to his brand-new baby gym and I like it because it's cool and dark under there, just us two. But I can't tell her that in case I sound deranged.

The easy chat works its magic though, strips away humiliation like old wallpaper, making me feel normal, so I'm really not prepared when she says it.

No fuss. No warning. She gives all 'her women' a score out of five for their pelvic-floor strength. Based on what she'd expect a woman to be six weeks post-birth, she'd give me — nearly three months post birth — minus three.

'*FUCK OFF,*' I think. MINUS THREE? I didn't know it was a test. If I'd known that, I would have revised. I don't get minus numbers. I got my photo in the local paper on A-Level results day. I want to do the test again and get an A.

What I actually say is worse. It's something like: 'No. Please. I can do better. Don't … Are you *writing it down*? Oh God! Don't write it down. Honestly, we can sort this out.'

And then, 'What does five mean? How do I get a five?'

I don't even explore how it feels to be one of 'her women'. A member of this exclusive broken pissy club. I don't want to be a bad loser but even though I don't understand the scoring minus three sounds disastrous, it implies not enough effort or skill.

She spots the fear, and showers me with quick reassurance. There is so much that we can improve. I'm young, only 30, and this is great, it means there's all to play for here.

'*It didn't feel great just now, being the youngest in the waiting room,*' I think. She's still talking though.

The score is just a baseline, and no, I'm not completely broken and, don't worry, this doesn't mean that I can never have another baby. That last thought is so casually tossed out that I don't know what to say. I'm glad, I think, that I can probably have more babies. But I'm alarmed it was ever a question. Perhaps this thing is really serious.

I stretch a smile to feign relief. Hooray! More babies! And then feel a sob catch in my throat. I'd disguise it as a cough, but I've just put my leggings back on and I don't want to pee myself again.

'Well, I suppose it could be worse,' I say, with only a tiny falter.

She looks at me hard and sighs. Like she's sorry that this is all such a mess. That I'm so broken. Maybe she's guessed how I'm feeling now I'm back here, a few corridors away from the scene of the crime, when I should be at baby massage. And that hint of kindness is *the worst*. I feel more exposed than I was with my knickers off. It's like she can see exactly how fragile I am squeezed into my nursing bra, with dirty hair and pre-baby make-up that no longer fits my face.

She adds that I have '30 per cent sensation'. I can't tell if this is good or bad. She sounds hopeful, though I'm only half listening now.

She says we can use 'conservative measures' and 'pelvic floor exercises'. We needn't worry about operations just yet. We can start 'bladder retraining', once I've filled in my 'bladder diary'.

She hands over some pamphlets. They all say 'bladder' on them. I finger the paper, scanning. Drinking. Measuring. Recording. I hear her words too: 'routine', 'biofeedback', 'order', 'lifts', 'traffic lights'. None of it makes any sense.

Questions swirl, but I can't ask them. I can't grab them from my slipping mind. I'm supposed to be somewhere else, enjoying my maternity leave, stitches dissolved, and this mad, bad birth all over. I breathe deep to ward off rising panic. I want to tell her that I'm too young, and too busy, for this bullshit. That even if I have got a broken fanny, my to-do list includes more important matters like developing a new social identity, losing two stone, and raising a human.

But it isn't her fault, so I do the only thing I can do: I smile super brightly, tie my cardigan round my waist and act like I can just carry on. Like I can say 'incontinent' and 'vaginal' and 'tear' and work out which size Tena Lady to buy.

I decide to thank her for her time and offer her my hand. We bungle as we try to shake though. This everyday touch is too awkward. It feels implausible and wrong: now I'm really embarrassed. But I rescue it. I tell her I'll fill in the diary and do my exercises. *Look!* I've written '3 x 10' on my pamphlets to remind me. I will report back next week a new woman, a braver woman. I almost salute her.

As the door shuts behind me, I look at the blue-grey vinyl floor and bite my lip, but it's too late. Tears escape and cling to my cheeks. I can't stop them, but I can't let anyone see me actually cry either. There's been too much sympathy today. So I look for the nearest toilet and run, faster than I've run since before I got pregnant and massive, which feels like a different lifetime. I smash into the cubicle, ignoring the trail of piss behind me and my wet socks and shoes.

'*How the hell did I get here?*' I think, as I crumple to the floor and slide down beside the U-bend. '*And what the very fuck will become of me?*'

Part One

PREGNANCY AND CHILDBIRTH

Chapter 1

Speaking up

L ife doesn't always turn out the way you expect it to. I had my first child at the start of social media when 'sharenting' was just beginning as a phenomenon. Though micro blogging and even instant photo filters weren't a thing back in 2007, there was still the growing expectation that all of us could (and should) live lives that could be transmitted to the world, in photographic vignettes that showed we were 'smashing it' at every turn.

My first birth didn't really play to the script. My body and mind stopped working, just at the point they were supposed to be coming into their prime. I walked out of the maternity ward, at the ripe old age of 30, with a collection of incontinence issues that would unfold, over the next decade, into an epic drama. My fanny collapse was caused by a combination of unexceptional but damaging injury, unusually bad luck and a family history of physical flexibility that I'd always thought was a good thing. My ability to do the splits in my teens just meant my muscles and ligaments were easily stretched out of shape, especially the ones in my pelvic floor designed to hold my bits up and in place. It also left me mentally fragile. I found out first hand why incontinence is one of the last medical taboos. And the most stubborn.

In a society that fears the signs of old age as much as old age itself, and is judgemental and aggressive in the face of weakness and fallibility, incontinence remains an unmentionable. It has to, because it holds a mirror up to those fears, daring to suggest that physical ruin may come to us all with its public spectacle of humiliation.

Incontinence affects women more than men, so it doesn't get the attention it deserves, not least as there's an insidious underlying suggestion that leaking is just the natural consequence of having been a woman for a long time. Whether through genuine ignorance or belligerence, medics, and women themselves, stick to an old lie that incontinence is a normal part of growing old. Something women just have to put up with, like wrinkles, mansplaining or John Humphrys.

This is true all over the world, causing a negative cascade of distress and negligence. Incontinence is so stigmatised, sufferers are often voiceless, marginalised or ignored. Too smothered by shame and embarrassment to think they deserve treatment, let alone go and get it. According to research from the NCT (National Childbirth Trust), in 2016 38 per cent of UK women with incontinence issues were too embarrassed to tell a health professional about it at all. Many don't even tell their partners or closest friends.

It took me a long time to understand what had happened to me. I've had to put the story together from hospital letters, blogs, memories and medical notes, and my frantic scribbles about charities working in this area, media representations of leaking, medical research and campaigns.

I found a lot of information saying people should and could get help. What I didn't find a lot of was people sharing their actual experience or commiserating frankly about the heartbreak, mess, cost and absurdity of it all.

And that is what I am trying to offer here. Snapshots of that time, of my thinking and experience, over the decade in which my privates became public embarrassments more than once. A decade where I was desperate to know I wasn't alone, that other people found this stuff difficult, were scared of treatment and worried about its impact on themselves, their babies, their love lives.

Recall wasn't always easy. Like many people who have a traumatic birth, I had flashbacks. But not to the birth: to its aftermath and my first (but not last) adult experience of standing in a puddle of my own wee. To a Saturday morning in high summer, when the sharp sunlight exposed my brokenness and a shower disguised neither the blood pouring down my legs, nor the growing pool of urine at my feet.

I stared at myself, transfixed – what was left of *me* in this 'new mother' body? What exactly had been broken? What would ever work again? Had I asked for this, by giddily approaching birth with too much optimism? By not knowing quite what I was getting myself into?

In one hour of pushing, I'd transformed myself from young healthy woman to decrepit, pissy trainwreck, but I'd lost far more than some elasticity or neat folds of skin. I'd lost my balance. Reeling from the body-shock, I was diagnosed with post-natal depression and described as 'traumatised'; doctors even called it 'PTSD'.

There's only one photograph from that morning that doesn't give the game away. Where we've cropped the blood and stitches and three faces stare at the camera. In the black and white print, people kindly say we – me, my husband and the baby – look nice, but I can see my eyes are scary. The only person who has seen the colour one said: 'Burn it, love, you look A THOUSAND YEARS OLD.'

But the bigger shock was the realisation that however much you need time to stand still so you can process a difficult event, life's momentum has its own ideas, especially where childbirth is concerned. It's the most brutal lesson of birth: the world spins on without you at a breathtaking clip, and your baby just keeps growing, impervious to your inability to hold your head together.

Looking at the wider cultural and historical picture around birth injuries and leaking made me outraged too – why *had* women put up with this shit for so long? Even though it has presumably been happening since Eve or one of her daughters had the first third-degree tear (or worse) and had to clear up the mess without Kegels (first published descriptions, 1948), or a tumble drier. Or anyone first got drunk, old, menopausal, injured or sick, which is a large proportion of the Old Testament.

Why hadn't more people cracked with the loneliness of embodying taboo? Whenever I brought it up, other women started telling me their own stories, or more commonly those of their mothers, grandmothers, aunts. These may have been proxy stories, like when people are 'asking for a friend'. But I could hear the truth. Incontinence stories were out there, everywhere, but could only be whispered, or hidden in plain sight behind a specific brand of raucous toilet humour – jokes about pads, and trampolines, and the funny faces we pull when trying to work those pelvic floors.

Take the traditional Celtic parody campfire song, 'Seven Old Ladies', a rude take on an eighteenth-century ballad 'Johnny's So Long At The Fair'. It's best known for its first line, *Oh, dear! What can the matter be? Seven old ladies stuck in the lavatory* and describes a series of unfortunate women stuck in the loo. There are hundreds of variants on the verses but incontinence gets several mentions – little Miss Murry rushing and arriving too late, Miss Moore who can't wait and pees on the floor. It seems women having toilet trouble is a tale as old as time, a part of our cultural fabric, and yet incontinence remains fraught and confusing. Cosy jokes mask real peril – stigma bubbling beneath the cracks in our veneer of civilisation, challenging our definition of what an acceptable body is.

Help is available. In the UK physios, doctors and specialist nurses can all offer a safe space of acceptance where nobody is made to feel like an idiot or a nuisance, and these services offer very good results, but the social issue stops people even rocking up. Because just saying it is fine to get help ignores the truth: that being incontinent is grim and most people think of it as a problem for smelly old ladies or outcasts.

And that is what made me want to start talking about it: fury at the myths and misogyny, and the hope that hearing they weren't alone would encourage someone, anyone, to feel less wretched and get help. I needed to point out that incontinence can usually be fixed, and that a good life is possible even if it can't. That there are economic benefits to helping the leaky amongst us get dry. And that we all need to grow up and start talking about it properly because it is the right thing to do and it might make millions of lives better. And also, somehow, make mine better too.

People often ask if I've always been confident talking about this stuff. I should be so lucky. My hand was forced. Thirty-year-old me, despite being ready to build a houseful of boys, would still have rather died than fart in public. Forty-year-old broken me has had to find a way of living with the risk.

Bodily functions weren't polite talk when I was growing up. Not just in my family but everywhere. Gender lines were clearly drawn. Spunk and little boys tinkling was funny. Girls should shh about crouching to pee, and other emissions were unspeakable. Period blood was blue liquid in adverts, and Tiny Tears taught a generation that the bodily functions of girls should be invisible. We should embrace the drudge of parenting but ensure nothing that emerged from our little holes is more taxing than the occasional splash of water.

Coming (un)clean and talking about my broken fanny in public wasn't something I'd always planned. I was born with a feminist roar but not a lack of embarrassment; I had to build up that Teflon 'Tena bravado' from scratch, starting so stressed out in Mothercare that I was leaking everywhere – face tear-streaked, shoes in a puddle, my maternity bra on the verge of smelling like yoghurt.

The end of summer 2007, a large babywear shop

I am in Mothercare. I am not here to buy booties or baby socks or a new pram. I lived the excitement and the thrill of all that. I'm here because I vaguely remember they have a section full of products to help clear up mummy-made mess – from squirting breastmilk to post-birth bleeding, and including what I really need right now, the extensive day-to-day equipment to stop leaking so badly I ruin my trousers every time I push my buggy up the curb.

I've been told I have a problem down there – and it is already making my brain a bit wonky. I have referral letters in my changing bag to speak to a counsellor from the birth trauma team and have physio sessions booked in. I feel overwhelmingly disgusting. It is so distressing and stressful to risk peeing if I try to carry my baby in a sling or do any of the things other mums seem to be doing.

I've been making do with the sanitary towels left gathering dust in my bathroom while I was pregnant, but I'm learning that they can't really handle pee, which doesn't drip steadily like menstrual blood, but pours thick and fast if the floodgates open. And that if they get drenched, they are likely to chafe or disintegrate.

I wheel my son through, past the kids' clothes, the plimsolls and sunhats, the breastfeeding tops and the fancy dress outfits, kidding myself I can handle it, until I see the potties and baby-wipes. They signal we are in the zone: the Mothercare aisle of shame. It's a shrine to absorbency. The shelves piled high with plastic packaging. Packaging in soothing blues and greens, with teardrops to represent urine flow and big bold letters shouting loud about masking odour and discretion.

There are cartons of fake knickers, pads for your bed, and massive maternity towels all hiding next to the nappies. I am new to this. I didn't realise there were so many nappies. Nappies in every conceivable size and shape, for girls and boys, for swimming and sleeping, for potties and pulling up, and for useless broken muffs like mine.

I think, 'Nappies, nappies, everywhere, even ones for me' and then burst into tears. It is dawning on me that this embarrassing unholy mess is not a short-term issue. It is going to require these pads, probably a new mattress, and a way of preventing myself from ever crying again as I realise, standing there, that anything more than the most graceful sob also makes pee escape.

I stand stock-still and hope my jeans will soak up enough to save my dignity and pray. Pray (even though I believe in nothing), that I'll be able to get out of the shop without bumping into anyone I know. That I can escape without leaving an actual puddle on the floor.

I want to howl. It isn't *fair*. Incontinence paraphernalia is expensive, uncomfy and I'm permanently terrified of accidents in public that broadcast my brokenness. Also, it feels like admitting my big fear, that I may be stuck like this forever, to engage with buying all the different brands and working out which are my best fit.

But it's too pressing. So I call my mum. She's visiting anyway and organises some supplies, like she did with tampons and pads when I started.

The next week I have used them all up (a bad sign) but I am still scared of shopping for them and that Mothercare will invoice me if I did leave a puddle, so my husband has to step up and go on a pad hunt.

Three minutes' walk from our house, three million light years from his comfort zone, a ramshackle local pharmacy becomes his haven. The elderly pharmacist steps in, to support a tired young man with a whole new universe of stigma to conquer. Between them, they work the full gamut of adult diapers and my husband becomes an expert. The pharmacist knows to be kind, to pretend he doesn't know who I am even when my prescriptions become more embarrassing over the years, with antidepressants and other continence aids, and how to gently manoeuvre my husband away from the wrong sorts of products. I'm not sure which of us is more relieved when we get to grips with online shopping. I know we are all saved.

I'd love to say I rose above unrealistic ideas about bodies and childbirth, refused to enter willingly into the shameful silence of a condition whose very name is synonymous with immorality, excess, lack of control. That I cheerfully assessed my pee flow as 'heavy' and felt no irony about throwing my continence products into a basket with my baby's. That I didn't absorb it like a personal failing. But no. I faltered in the face of it all, regressing to a toddler state and letting someone else buy my nappies.

It seems completely ridiculous to be felled at the first hurdle, by a mishap in Mothercare, but perhaps it just exemplifies the way we never grow out of our primal fear of humiliation. We all remember *that* girl in the front row of assembly, too scared to put up her hand, an amber pool spreading out from under her short grey skirt. As an adult, repeating that image under strip lighting sent me into a spiral of self-hate. I had not been good enough at birth. I was being punished for becoming a hot sweaty mess and not channelling enough yoga or positive thinking. But that was madness talking – and conditioning.

For millennia, we've told women their bits are nasty and they shouldn't talk about them. And we've ridiculed, brutalised and excluded men and women who can't keep their pee or poo in place, despite the fact we all have bodies and know that bodies can break, and incontinence is widespread.

It is hard to properly understand why something so common and blatantly grim isn't treated with more seriousness and kindness. And why even when we do talk about it we can't rise above silly jokes or fear; these both blur the landscape and mean patients can't make meaningful choices about their care.

I set out to search for the root causes and to work out what it was in my early experiences, or even in all of our early experiences, that keeps us locked in the little girls' room imagining we don't deserve any better than walking around with a creaking mattress between our thighs, and jeans that need washing every time we go dancing.

There must be some common threads that created the perfect storm of shame and confusion around continence. Something in our fabric has led us to a point where an often-curable condition is suffered in upset silence. I was lonely but I was never alone. One in three women experiences incontinence in her life, but thousands and thousands never even try to get treatment. Even those that do take years to summon the courage. Feeling personal shame at wetting oneself is understandable, but for a whole society to shame sufferers? That is *bullshit*.

We can't leave continence languishing in the half-light of humour and metaphor. We must change the landscape. And perhaps we can start by talking more clearly about bodies, vaginas, menstruation, childbirth, and reassuring women that when those things go wrong, they are allowed to 'make a fuss' about it.

I'd love to say it all began for me staring at a box of continence pads and realising we can all do better than this – but stories, like social conditioning, never start where you think.

For me, the seeds go back to what I learned about my body growing up, and being in a generation taught to find our clitoris but given scant info on our pelvic floor. It is accelerated by living in the digital age as I mature, where women's bodies are still endlessly up for public description and criticism, but where their voices are characterised as rebellious, frightening, unreliable, and hysterical. And it's complicated by the war of ideas beginning amongst women themselves, as we try to work out how to give each other honest body knowledge, without scaring or pigeon-holing anyone with the truth about childbirth – the good, the empowering, and the slightly more ugly.

The seeds also go back, very specifically for me, to my own denial; my squeamishness about my own body and my inability to understand how it would or wouldn't work when performing basic reproductive functions.

Take the weeks leading up to my thirtieth birthday. Fat, furious and fecund, I found these fantasies and contradictions about women and bodies had turned my mind off completely, and my main concerns were only how to change a nappy on a little boy and what sort of novel I should write on maternity leave. I knew, due date looming, that I was standing on a precipice, but I was busy planning how quickly I could get back to being me again, ignoring the strong possibility that, however it worked out, I was going to be changed by the experience forever.

Chapter 2

Childbirth – Expectations

My understanding of childbirth was, at best, top-line when I first became pregnant. For all my feminist posturing, I knew that sometimes there was *damage*, and that some older ladies had 'no control'. What I didn't know, or perhaps more correctly didn't appreciate fully, was that it was possible that these kind of rank medical realities could soon become my own.

I was exactly the *wrong* kind of over-informed.

For example, I spent a lot of time reading the bits of pregnancy books that tell you which size of fruit or vegetable your foetus corresponds to week-by-week. I could win pub quizzes in it. At work we nicknamed these grape-to-melon journeys *In Fruitero* and *Fruits of the Womb*. I pushed the more terrifying information about actually hoofing a giant fruit out of my teeny hole to the back of my mind along with piles, varicose veins and all the novels I'd read where childbirth ended in disaster. I really was not ready to give birth.

Early June 2007, a pretty garden, full of pregnant women past the point of no return

It is a momentous but scary day. It's not my due date – I'm not worried about *that* – it's the 'women only' afternoon at my antenatal class.

We are all around 36 weeks – almost at term (aka pumpkin). The session is for expectant mothers to ask any questions that

Baby Growth Size

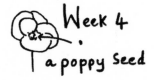 **Week 4**
a poppy seed

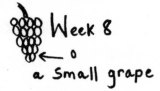 **Week 8**
a small grape

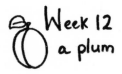 **Week 12**
a plum

Week 16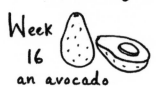
an avocado

Week 20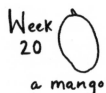
a mango

Week 24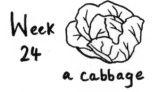
a cabbage

Week 28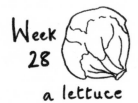
a lettuce

Week 32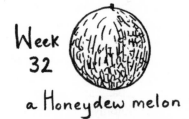
a Honeydew melon

Week 36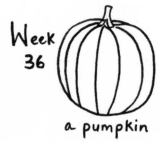
a pumpkin

Week 40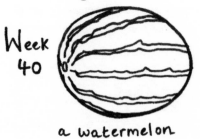
a watermelon

they don't want to voice in front of other people's partners. These turn out to be about excessive watery discharge (rank, but okay), cervical mucus plugs (oh GOD), bloody or meconium-tinged waters (not nice or okay, because it means the baby is pooing inside you), pain (shhh), haemorrhoids (yuck) and pooing after giving birth (apparently a massive *thing*, as in a milestone, and a massive thing, as in 'like a log'). All the totally grim shit, basically. I can barely listen.

The church hall we normally use for classes is booked, so we are in one of the pregnos' garden. I stare into its lovely pond as birth injuries and rare post-birth nightmares are discussed around me: stitches, post-natal depression and postpartum psychosis.

These things sound awful. They make me feel nearly as uncomfortable as the hand or foot reaching right down into my cervix. I let out a groan.

It is a strange situation. I feel like we are playing at being grown-ups. We're still discussing what slippers we want to wear in labour. I suspect that what most of us really want to know is this: 'Will we shit ourselves in childbirth? How much? And how can we avoid it?'

Our antenatal teacher instructs us to buy a sieve if we want a water birth, which doesn't bode well, and I'm considering asking if there's a way to con midwives into giving us enemas, like in the good old days, to avoid this happening.

I do have one question, but I am scared to ask it. I have heard a throwaway remark about episiotomies, from someone who has already had a baby and around whom I now feel like a credulous teen. An episiotomy is a cut made to make the entrance/exit of the vagina bigger. Like enemas, it was a common procedure in the '70s and '80s but only usually happens now with instrumental deliveries or very large babies. My friend made it sound as if her episiotomy was 'performed' with scissors. This would make me cross my legs if my firm, space-hopper belly was not resting between them. I steel myself and ask it very quickly, hoping to hear that supersized openings are seamlessly and painlessly encouraged by unicorns.

An Episiotomy

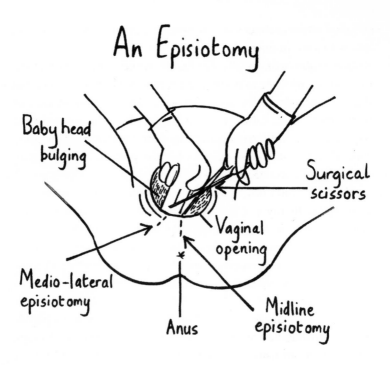

Baby head bulging

Surgical scissors

Vaginal opening

Medio-lateral episiotomy

Anus

Midline episiotomy

'Yes, we use scissors,' says the teacher, who has also worked as a midwife. 'What did you think we used?'

I only think, 'Oh fuck.'

If I'm honest I am a bit scared and embarrassed by the whole session. It feels like we are tempting fate by talking about difficulties and problems, and I'm not the only one wincing at the word 'perineum' (of which more in Chapter 6) and the suggestion that some people stretch it with almond oil. And it seems a bit pointless to hear about the dangers now – I can't exactly back out.

As the session wraps up, our teacher tries very hard to tell us about pelvic floor exercises and how to do them. I smile, smugly. I can stop my pee mid-flow, so I guess I'm okay. (I later find that stopping your pee to check your control is no longer recommended due to infection risks – so don't try it at home, kids.)

I don't want to think about squeezing though, I want to go and inhale Soleros in the park.

Our leader womanfully continues, using a metaphor about lifts pulling up floor to floor, and tells us to try them. There and then. I look around the table and see a faraway look in each of the women's eyes. I don't see that look again, that contraction of concentration and gurning surprise, until I'm potty-training my son, when it instils utter panic as I know it means he's about to crap on the floorboards.

That's the only time I remember the subject of incontinence coming up in my pregnancy, apart from the ominous pads suggested for my hospital bag. I try to make the lift metaphor work but I just can't get the knack. So I shelve the thought, and start looking forward to next week. That will be our last session when we get to hear what positions we need to be in to give birth.

I do actually master kickass Kegels years later, when a physio tells me to imagine I am trying to adjust a slightly not-in-enough tampon without using my fingers and I think 'BINGO!' But by then I've also realised the truth of what birth can become, and how accurate bodily metaphors can be.

My post-birth body was the best metaphor for mothering ever. Proof that there had been, and would forever be, a ravaging of everything: my vagina, my personal space, my bookshelves, my dining room, my tits. All of them stretched and pulled into a new beginning by a magical creature tearing his way out. How could I have been so ignorant of what was to come?

I didn't expect my birth to be so awful because I had studiously ignored the potential for childbirth to be crazy, horrific, boring and seemingly endless for my entire life. I didn't think it would be easy or beautiful or empowering, I just didn't expect the hip-rocking explosion that destroyed my body and sense of self. Or such an epic clean-up job afterwards. Women are supposed to be good at mess, right? But the task overwhelmed me.

My most firmly entrenched ideas about giving birth came from the births I'd 'seen' myself – on screen, or in novels and poems – although even then I cherry-picked what I could bear to believe. I became addicted to TV births while I was pregnant. Real and fictional journeys of new life in simple, narrative forms beginning with a hopeful bump and ending with a baby. Most of them were romanticised or overdramatised and skimped on the more mundane details, and the aftermath.

It wasn't until 2012 (too late for me!) when *Call the Midwife* started sneaking radical feminism onto Sunday night TV that I saw anything suggesting that the birthing experience, like the pregnancy belly, continues after you leave the delivery suite. The drama's plots, inspired by a midwife's memoirs, explore the up- and downsides of birth and reproduction as part of a woman's whole life, from dangerous illegal abortions to sepsis, through incontinence, birth trauma, adoption, prolapse, bleeding out, maternal stroke and depression.

To be fair to *Call The Midwife*, it showed other less dramatic but important aftermath scenarios too, giving us new women every week: mothers who were lonely, mothers who were happy, mothers who were relieved, mothers who survived, mothers who were traumatised, mothers stricken with grief, mothers who were empowered. Nice women, bad women, happy women. Crucially, such stories point out that birth transforms everything, so it is almost impossible to spring back into your world unchanged like a soap opera character, a lesson that might have helped that first-time-pregnant me.

The landscape of fiction offers us versions of ourselves, ideas of who we could or should (or shouldn't) be. They are not real life, but these templates drip drip drip into our minds by stealth, giving hope, alongside entertainment, but also encouraging a dreamy attachment to lives we cannot actually live.

One channel had a baby hour when I was pregnant, which I watched devoutly. And when Abby in *ER* had her awful premature labour, I howled on the sofa until my husband offered (begged?) to turn it off.

'Noooooo!' I wailed, hiccupping into the screen. 'If you turn it off I'll (*hic*) never (*shudder*) know (*deep breath*) what (*shuddering deep breath*) happens!'

I'd been watching *ER* as woman and girl; these characters had seen me through relationships, singledom, co-habiting, marriage and now this, my first confinement.

There are studies on how the traumatic nature of TV and film births contributes to birth fear amongst expectant mothers. For me, I suspect, despite Abby's horrific birth, the opposite was true. I still secretly based my birth fantasies on Daphne's fully-clothed roadside delivery from *Neighbours*. When births looked really scary, I just switched off my brain and focused on the next episode or instalment where all was well again.

It wasn't that I hadn't heard any birth stories before, but the details were often sketchy, perhaps because people self-edit so as not to scare the pregnant woman, or any woman come to that. And also because births can be strange, drugged-up, time-hopping affairs, and their retelling difficult. How do you explain something that's messy, medical, natural, emotional, linear, episodic, physical, dreamlike, religious, boring, peaceful, frightening, easy and difficult all at once?

When I was a child my mother had given me, rightly, because I was so young, edited descriptions of her births. Babies just pop out, she said, no fuss, not like the scary births on *EastEnders* or *Brookside*, full of screaming and emergencies. I learned my mum's stories by heart. Her waters going twang with me. Twins nearly arriving in the car one frosty April morning. My middle sister flying out like Supergirl with her hand outstretched. They thrilled me because they were so exciting and happy. I didn't ask for more detail, ever, and happily ran with these family snapshots right up to my own labour.

Now I wish I'd known more. We may have been brought up to laugh at the women of old who didn't have *Sex and the City* or, later, *Girls* to help them talk about our sexual parts frankly. We might even think ourselves better for our girl power fuelled talk of orgasms, G-spots (remember those?), cunnilingus and *The Vagina Monologues*. But they, our grandmothers and theirs, at least had the sense to talk about birth properly to each other, even if it was behind closed doors. Well, those that survived it.

And they'd attended births too, or heard the hoo-ha. They didn't rock up entirely unprepared. Not like me: one minute a career woman on the brink of having it all, with a swollen bellyful of son, a polite if vague birth plan (I didn't want to be bossy, or act like an expert) and hopes for an uneventful water birth, and the next: BAM! Broken.

I know some people who felt awfully cheated and angry with the world because nobody told them the truth. My anger was more about getting broken bits along with bunches of flowers as my induction to motherhood. But the truth had been out there, so perhaps I'd just ignored it, favouring the sugar-coated ideas I'd swallowed as a child.

The week before I gave birth, my mum told me that she had had to bite down on a cloth during the worst of it, a soft modern bit between her teeth. But my shell had hardened by then, though I did follow in her footsteps and bite down on a gas and air mouthpiece so hard I cracked a molar right down to the root.

However, when I have some distance to analyse what has happened to me, I realise with surprise that when I was pregnant someone did give me an example of a film that showed the visceral realities of childbirth, and in technicolour too. That person was a workplace friend, who I met fresh from her birth centre experience when I was around five months.

March 2007, a London street, pretending I'm not in denial

It is a bright wintery day and I have a foetus the size of a large mango hidden in my midi-bump. My colleague Cat has popped into work on her maternity leave and we've had lunch. We are engrossed in a conversation about childbirth, ignoring the looks we get every time we say 'vagina' in the street. I've had a scan and know it is a boy, which makes me feel adult and almost confident.

Cat has given me vivid snippets of her water birth, including references to tears, stitches, internal examinations, fat-fingered midwives and a spinal block. Even though she has told me so much, I sense she's skirted something. And that she knows I'm clinging to squeamishness like a life raft. Nevertheless, there's a thrill. It's like being back at school, fantasising about what it's like to be a grown-up. Then Cat stops on the pavement and bravely cuts through the angst. She stares at me, perhaps seeing how scared and ill-prepared I really am, and says she needs to tell me something another woman told her when she was at the point of no return. I am so terrified it will be about shitting that I nearly burst into tears.

It is worse.

'You know how people keep saying giving birth was the best day of their life? That it is amazing? And that they enjoyed it? You know it is okay if it isn't the best day of your life, right? And if you don't enjoy it? Giving birth. I mean, it was amazing to have my baby and I loved him and everything, but it wasn't really the best day of my life, Luce. It's okay if it isn't. Lots of women don't like it. You don't have to feel pressure to enjoy it.'

It feels so startlingly true that it makes my head rock. I glance at my bump, not yet stretch-marked, already bullet-shaped. I grasp at the moment's courage and, closing my eyes, I voice out loud the proper question, the real question I should ask someone, and resolve to believe the answer.

'What was it like then?' I say quickly. 'What was it actually like, giving birth in the water?'

'*Jaws*,' she says, without hesitation. 'It was like *Jaws*.' Fade to black.

Summer 2007, the last chance for knowledge: a church hall full of women at 'term' and their wild-eyed partners

We're back in the church on a nylon carpet with Mary and Joseph looking over us. Our antenatal class teacher has invited us to act out a mock C-section, thankfully without props, but it feels a bit rude, given Mary's experience in the straw.

The teacher gives us a roll call of how many people are likely to be in the room if we need a Caesarean, and how they will support us. I think of poor young Mary on her own in a barn, squatting amongst the droppings. I hope Joseph was the sort of guy who held her hand, not one who turned slightly greenish, and that the inn keeper's wife told her she was brave and helped cut the cord. It feels silly to be acting out an operation, but it will help later. Not because I remember any particular details, but because having seen exactly how many people are likely to be staring up your chuff when someone hits an alarm bell, that one part of labour at least isn't a shock.

We talk about birth positions and act them out too. This is as excruciating as it sounds. We are too far gone in the grimness of pregnancy to pat each other on the back and mime contractions. Sensing our disquiet, our teacher shows us a series of diagrams on worksheets. One involves sitting on a chair the wrong way, looking over the back of it – cowboy style. It's called 'upright forward and open' or 'UFO' – after the position in which it puts the pelvis. It seems alien to me. Our teacher, who is acting each one out, adds that it works just as well on the toilet.

'Jesus Christ,' I think. 'Sitting on the fucking loo?!'

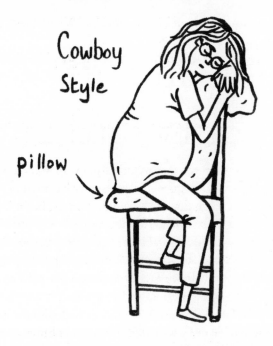

Cowboy Style

pillow

The next week, I meet another pregnant woman, now on her third baby. 'Oh yes,' she says, when I confide my horror. 'I spent hours on the loo. It was the only place I could get comfortable.'

I imagine myself astride a loo, as if it is a horse and the cistern is the neck I am clinging to. I find that image revolting, me straining on a toilet as if my baby is a massive poo. And what if the baby falls in? I don't want my husband to see me like that. Riding the toilet like a horse. *That* would be the most undignified thing ever.

Chapter 3

Childbirth – Reality

I spend the first few hours of my labour sitting on a toilet, groaning and riding it like a horse. This is the most dignified moment of that sordid 19 hours, probably of the following two years too.

The entire process from start to finish is a catalogue of shock, boredom and humiliation. The first thing I do when it is over is text Cat with no weight, name or details, just the line: 'IT'S A FUCKING CONSPIRACY.'

As I should have expected, my conspiracy involves screaming, mooing, begging and whimpering, with side orders of physical degradation and waiting around – though, unexpectedly, I do crack a couple of rude but well-timed jokes.

When I try to recall any more than that immediately afterwards, the screen fades to white and then I'm standing in front of a mirror by the horse-toilet, which is in a shower room off the labour ward, dominated by a large mirror, clearly installed by some kind of sadist. There I stand, a crazy ghostlike version of myself, staring at a deflated, bloated parody of my sweet, sweet rounded pregnant body, blood on my knees, pee and blood flowing down from the gap between my wobbling legs. Under a warm shower, I find no comfort. The shock of how little is left of my privates is underscored when I use Original Source shower gel and it smarts like motherfuck. But those things are nothing on my face, at once as beautiful, young and glowing as a brand-new moon, and as old and bitter and angry as time.

The heat and steam and rusty smells rise. My senses are electric. I can hear a midwife outside nearly as loudly as I can hear my own heart, thudding under the weight of love for my son. Not a love that rushes in, a giddy flow, an excitement, but something that transcends time and binds us, like skin fusing back together after a burn. The midwife sounds worried but I can't place her concern. I'm scared she is going to tell me off. Perhaps she's worried I've been in there too long, or I'm using up all the hot water; perhaps the door that was sticking hasn't shut properly and she's worried about the bloody lake (half piss, half what is left behind), seeping into the corridor and alarming some poor wretch on their way in. She asks if I need help. I don't know if I need it, or what that would look like. I'm splitting. I don't want anybody, ever, to witness the state I am in. But I want very much for someone to touch me to remind me that I'm human.

When I finally do remember what happened before that, it isn't very nice.

July 2007, *tired maternity wing, large teaching hospital*

I am in labour. When it starts, 15 minutes after my husband got on the tube to work, I find that ironic. As it progresses, I forget what 'ironic' means, along with my name, everything I've ever learned, and my sense of being a person anchored in time.

We arrive mid-morning, and I'm told I'm three or four centimetres dilated, and 'doing well'. It is up to me whether we stay or go home. My Facebook status, a novelty in 2007, is 'Luce Brett is in labour.' I feel quite violently paranoid that if I go home I will have failed publicly at giving birth. I'll have shown myself up as a wuss, and someone unable to follow instructions.

We decide to stay.

We're told the baby is back-to-back, which means he's the wrong way round and will come out 'face-to-pubes' if he doesn't turn. I shudder at this and spend several hours contracting and trying to talk him round.

Night comes and the midwives send my husband home. The labour ward is busy now, they say, and as I'm only 1cm further on, I'm 'wasting' a room.

They shuttle me to a communal ward-cum-corridor and tell me I can get some sleep. This isn't true. There's no rest here – not between the noisy labouring women, poorly women, screeching babies, and the staff shouting 'Shhh' and telling me off for whimpering when the gas and air runs out.

I pack my bag and notes between wrenching contractions, and offer to go home. I know my husband would hate the 'business end' but he would at least be nice. A doctor rolls his eyes, and tells me I have to stay. I feel chastised. I'm in dilation no man's land. Too slow for labour ward, too speedy and in pain for this hellhole. And I have no one to help me. Not even as my entire world turns to shit in the most disgusting toilet I have ever seen.

I think of *Trainspotting* as I lurch in there the first time, ignoring the night staff tutting. The toilet would win a BAFTA for grime.

At first, I think it isn't *that* dirty, just old, and tarnished, with a dripping tap. Though there is loo roll all over the floor and paper towels, some used, overflowing from the bin. A light flickers and buzzes; another one doesn't work at all. There are boxes of Lucozade bottles in the corner for diabetes tests. I toy with pinching one (I'm not virtuous, even in childbirth) but I'm scared of getting into even more trouble. And I don't know if I should drink anything as I can't really wee properly, even though I'm bursting.

I manage a trickle but it really hurts. I go back to bed, steadying myself on the wall of the corridor. Then I need a wee again.

This carries on for two hours. Clambering on and off hospital beds and high toilets. The night feels dangerous. And with each trip I am fascinated but scared by the shapes and sounds my body is making. I groan and huff, and push the walls. I lumber. My belly is taut. It's heavy too, solid. I'm pushing back inside me. My back is curving. My legs buckle.

On the final trip, I sit on the loo and stare at the dripping tap, the horrid hot water dispenser, the filthy-looking walls covered in stickers, commands about cleanliness, demands for washing. I am about to laugh at the irony, but I'm fumbling for the word, when suddenly I lunge.

I fall forwards, making an enormous guttural EUURRRRGHHHHH sound. I can't tell if I lose consciousness. I do a full lurching body spasm: I strain, am sick, wet myself, and, I think, shit myself too. As I wake, there is warm liquid all over my legs and thighs. Blood? Wee? My waters? My waters with blood or wee in it? I can't tell in the dim light. It just all looks brown-ish.

I spit out as much of the sick as I can and start to try and mop up the mess. Crawling round, acid hair stinging my eyes, cracking lips. I use paper towels and scrub the floor, hoping to God that at least some of the shit is mine, and none of it belongs to my baby: because my brain is kicking in through the panic and I know that if my waters are full of meconium, that first shit they do, it is a bad sign. If the baby has pooed before it has even come out, that means it is distressed.

I think, 'You and me both, kiddo.'

It's too dark to clear up a mess like this and I start to crawl back to the bed and the light. It must be safer there.

I've heard people say it is good if women talk to their babies in labour.

'Maybe we'll die here, me on all fours, you half out, both of us in a toilet, covered in shit,' I nearly whisper to my son. Instead, I say out loud 'please don't die' as the pain ramps up, making me nauseous. It doesn't feel like a good or productive pain, it just feels stuck.

When I get to the bed, I'm shaking. I want to rant at the two women at the nurses' station who watched me crawl the full distance. 'Perhaps they didn't see us,' I hope, but for survival's sake, I do something far more shameful. I start to beg.

Apologies cascade out of me: 'Sorry. Sorry. Please help me. I think my waters have broken. I'm so sorry. I think there might be meconium in it. I think I wet myself. I couldn't clean it all up. There's still poo on the floor in there. Please help us. Please. I'm sorry.'

A midwife runs, from somewhere. She's not ignoring me like the other staff seem to have been doing. She's my defender. She injects pethidine in my leg, but as the next contractions hit, I start shouting. I actually put the hand that isn't gripping the bedrail over my mouth to try and stop the noises bellowing out, but I can't.

The sound is so awful that my husband can hear me in the background when the midwives ring to tell him to come back in. His first words when he arrives are 'What the hell have you done to her?'

In the labour ward, I am now 8.5cm. Though perhaps I am misremembering the 0.5. I am super speedy now in any case. I scream. My eyes roll. I am possessed. Growling. Heaving. Shrieking. I'm Jamie Lee Curtis in *Halloween* and Linda Blair in *The Exorcist*. A midwife tells me she is worried about my throat.

'I'm worried about my cunt,' I reply.

The midwife ignores my potty mouth, but writes in my notes that I am 'extremely distressed' and they agree to do an epidural.

So instantaneous is the effect that I offer to go down on the female anaesthetist who performs it. Later, I think there's some kind of spinal block too though I lose track of what's being done. All I know for certain is I want everything: I don't care anymore. I have a catheter now, snaking out between my legs and tubes plugged into my hands. And then I realise it. I'm not shouting anymore. There's silence.

'See, a different woman,' says an experienced midwife as she hands me over to a student called Kay. I'm calm, chatty even, trippy. We listen to The Beatles on our new iPod as morning breaks. That's enough to save us. My husband sings and holds me. We pretend nothing bad has happened and hope for the best. In an hour I'm a perfect 10 (cm dilated), and in the perfect insult, my epidural is turned off for pushing. I am about to express my annoyance about losing pain relief at this, the worst bit, but life beats me to it and … BAM! We're back in the Somme.

Blood pumps from my hand because I've wrenched my cannula out somehow. People keep appearing. Rushing in and out. I see the doctor who told me off. He's nice now and looks concerned. The smells and the tacky feel of everything are extraordinary. The room is so bright, clear and loud, I can almost hear my skin split.

Two gloved hands go between my legs and are lifted up, ruby red with my blood. I think they belong to another doctor, an older woman, but I've lost track. She leans in with some scissors then withdraws, says they won't bother with an episiotomy (the size of my hole isn't the problem anymore because I've already torn it more than they would cut – Go, Luce!) but they will still use a ventouse (a vacuum sucker) if I don't push the baby out in the next few minutes because our baby's heart is beating too fast. It's a competition now. We're on the clock.

Kay looks conspiratorially up through the V of my bent knees and speaks directly to me, ignoring the drama around us. I can feel her breath on my thighs. 'You can do this on your own, Luce. I know you can,' she urges in a loud whisper.

I close my eyes and push as a pool of warm blood forms on the large square absorbent sheet she has whisked under my bum.

But it isn't just drama. At the same time, it is kind of serene. It's 9 a.m. in July and I can feel the warm sun on my left cheek, and smell someone smoking outside. I don't mind. I quite fancy a fag myself right now. A fag and a cup of tea and to just watch the movement and the people coming in. Are they prepping for something else? A C-section? Forceps? I don't care. I just want this to finish. To be over. I'm doing exactly what I'm told to do by Kay because she's the only one using my name.

Later, Kay tells me she was proud of me for being so stoical and brave through the pushing, especially with the tear. She congratulates me. I daren't shatter the illusion and tell her I simply assumed we were both dying, me and him. And I didn't care. That's bravery for you.

And then wow! He's born. I touch his head as he is crowning, after refusing a mirror to look. I don't want to, but Kay takes my hand and pulls it down between my legs. She says it will help, and she's right. It does. His head is bumpy and weird and familiar all at once. And warm and wet amongst the tangle of my bloody pubes. The inside is coming out. I can feel he's nearly there and give it a last guttural scream.

For years to come, I will put my palm over the top of his head to check, yes, it still feels the same, has the same shape. It's a comfort and I'm sad when he is seven and I can't make out the contours in the same way anymore, even when I sneak a kiss and stroke his hair while he's asleep.

He's so beautiful my world stops and life throws me back into the room, choking, because I have no choice, and he's lifted and passed up to me. I think I might vomit. I don't know what to say to him.

I can't say what I am thinking, which is 'Shit! What have we done?' I want him to hear something important. This is our Mothercare Moment after all.

I look down at him, his tiny shoulders, heather-coloured and hot on my chest, and whisper: 'Hello, little one.'

Kay is coaxing out the ragged afterbirth and I think I'm quite sick. There are tubes and bowls of blood everywhere. I slur my words. My legs shake. My husband takes his top off and lets the naked boy lie skin-to-skin over his daddy's heartbeat. We tell family but my mind is flitting.

I think, 'Fucking hell! William Blake was underselling it in "Infant Sorrow"' and snatch a line I learned in primary school from somewhere:

My mother groan'd! my father wept. / Into the dangerous world I leapt

But also, back in the room I think: 'Why do all these people keep cocking their heads to the side and looking at something?'

I realise later they are assessing the damage, looking for an experienced enough midwife to stitch me up; at the time they look like weird mimes.

Kay dresses our boy and sings him 'Happy Birthday'. I realise I don't even know the date, but I can't crack despite this disconnection because for a moment, with her voice and that tune, for one perfect moment, the room enjoys the everyday magic trick of birth. We all breathe the beauty of a furious creature, screaming his reedy scream, changing the make-up of the whole world forever by being born.

I think, 'At least it is over.'

The next afternoon, too early probably, we stagger out into the natural light, which seems changed, and become the clichéd couple arguing over a car seat. We scrabble and panic, inept in the face of too many straps and safety warnings. My hands shake but I don't matter anymore. I'm tearful, incoherent. I can't remember if he's a boy or a girl. I don't know what anyone told me, or whether I'm still in trouble with the nurses. When he's strapped in and shouting and we are ready to leave, I say:

'It's going to be fine, now, isn't it? It's going to be okay, right?'

'Yes,' says my husband. 'We don't ever have to go back there again.'

Chapter 4

Coming home

The following day, July 2007, a lounge full of flowers and presents

Our very favourite people meet our boy that afternoon. I'm still in my maternity tunic but I smile for the cameras and we worship his perfect shiny feet. He's glowing with life and somehow so are we.

My parents, only just 50, bring one of their old uni friends down to their first meeting. He visited me in hospital when I was born in 1977 and it feels so right. A different first-time family together again. My sisters kiss their nephew on the lips in turn as he closes his eyes and scowls at all of us. My mum asks about my stitches, but I don't know where to start, especially in the middle of so much love and happiness, so I give fragments of the nastiness but mostly say I'm 'a bit sore' and resolve to make the best of the things that are already starting to go right.

I don't need to learn to breastfeed as my son does it for us. My luck comes in with my milk. He latches with vigour and precision immediately, ferocious enough to make the let-down pain last just seconds. My mum winces as he attacks his way on and tells me that I was the same. On my baby hospital notes, a midwife wrote 'good little sucker', she remembers. There's a joke in there somewhere.

My stitches do heal quickly, my tummy starts dropping back; the only thing is I'm always weeing into my pants. I am repeatedly told this is normal. The family have left and we're on the verge of hospital sign-off when something terrible happens.

I'm feeding in the kitchen, surrounded by cooled boiled water and olive oil, which we've been told to use instead of wipes, and I get a lurching urge to push. It's weird, painful. I'm scared I'll drop the baby. I make the animal noise I made in the toilet, a sort of prehistoric moo, and then all these blood clots start falling out of me.

The lochia, the period-style bleed after you give birth, has been quite gross, but these are big oily lumps that slide out of my hands like chicken giblets. I crawl upstairs to the bathroom, trying to contain them. There's blood on the carpet though.

I think, 'my poor landing'.

We ring the labour ward. They are very, very nice to me this time. I have to describe the clots with domestic comparisons – not a dinner plate, no, but yes, an apple, bigger, but flatter, not as round.

'It looks like sundried tomatoes,' I add, helpfully, always with the foodstuffs. But I really don't feel very well.

They readmit us both. We have matching wristbands. As we haven't registered him yet, my son doesn't officially exist. He's still me. They tell me to sleep, but I am back in the ward with the horrible toilet and Lucozade, listening to other women howl all night. This time, at least, I have my own room, 'for privacy'. In that room, doctors, midwives and students troop in to look, hourly, at how bloody my sanitary pads are, weigh them and check if there are more lumps of placenta left up there. They give examinations, with commentaries, for the hoards. One shows my husband a clot of mine that has got caught on a speculum. I'd run away but I am attached to a drip.

I think, 'At least my baby is in a plastic cot rather than halfway out of my vagina'.

They let us go but say we must come back immediately if it happens again, preferably bringing some of the clots with us.

I think '*Seriously?*' But when it does happen again I dutifully collect it all in an ice-cream tub.

Another day back in the ward and I feel cheated. Cheated that I am missing all the visitors and fun. I want to show my boy off, not lie in hospital with a cannula.

The third time it happens I get a new panic. Maybe I am making a fuss. No one expected it to happen again, that's why I didn't have the op to clear me out. I can't tell any more: am I dying, or failing? Or just making a massive meal out of something 'natural' that happens to all women?

I show the third clots to my mum and my teenage sister who have come down to visit again. My mum, who has had four babies, says we need to go to hospital, NOW.

My sister adds, 'Don't ever show me anything that rank again!'

I refuse the ambulance the midwife wants to send, as it feels too awkward. I don't know if it's exhaustion or returning to the hospital but I'm so distressed about more nights on that ward that the sympathetic doctor who observes me agrees I can wait for my blood results at home.

When we get home, I sneak to the toilet because I can't think of anywhere else to hide. My privates have been on parade for days now, I know there's little left to preserve, but I can't face the world.

My husband breaks my heart with his efforts to normalise everything. He's put all the sanitary gubbins in a basket on the window shelf and washed the walls and floor after the last big bleed. It smells of love and Flash.

It's the first few minutes I've been in a room on my own with no one touching my body since the awful shower after birth. Alone is nice. I hurt, but today has been victorious. We've escaped the ward. We're home. Downstairs, the baby squalls. I twinge with missing him, but still I hide. The volume rises.

My husband comes up and knocks on the door. He doesn't mean to follow me around but we are all new to this and our son is not bothering to filter his annoyance that he has such incompetent, shaky fools to take care of him.

My husband knocks again. He knows I'm scared, but the baby's screaming now.

I let them in and my son latches greedily onto my breast like the mammal he is as I still sit on the pan. He closes his eyes and sucks, emitting little earnest sighs as his belly swells, tummy to Mummy. Tears resting like forgotten jewels on his peach-skin cheeks. I look up to my husband's face. We've done it. We've stopped the crying. This dysfunctional display is a victory of sorts. Maybe we can move on from birth drama and leave the bogs of shame forever.

I look up. From the corner of my eye, I can see quite clearly a bloody handprint on the door frame.

Late July 2007, *waiting for the midwife sign-off*

I remain a patient for weeks. The baby's fine. Furious, but luminous in glorious summer. The community midwives still pop in every other day though they are surely tired of our story by now. I don't know what the first three weeks after a spontaneous vaginal delivery should be like control-wise, but I do know I can't really walk upstairs without a warm rush of weeing.

I try to talk to them about my fanny feeling broken and wrong, but they assure me the leakiness should stop soon. Mainly they seem so impressed that we haven't completely imploded, that I think they put it down to shock.

I feel wobbly in other ways too; the baby hasn't slept for more than two hours in a row yet, and when he does sleep, he likes to be absolutely certain that I am awake. But everyone says I've had a horrible time and it is normal to be unsettled, tearful and spaced out. I'm not sure though. I'm beginning to narrate my life in my head as if I don't really exist in the real world …

Early August 2007, kitchen, evening, a radio plays
'Here Comes The Sun'

The song fills the air: it *is* like a movie. You remember singing through contractions in the nice bit of your labour when your husband came back. Corny youngsters on the precipice of something you didn't understand, singing and coaxing him out.

Is it real? Did you dream it? You ask your husband if he remembers and he holds your face and says, 'Of course I do.'

Maybe there is hope for you yet. It feels like a good moment that could change the course of everything.

And then it lands. A tidal wave of sadness. It hits, as you have been told, in the way tsunamis do: a wall of water, crashing into you, full submersion without the baptismal relief of rising again. You nearly lose your balance. You know now, you *know*, that no amount of jokes and good moments will stop you feeling like the world has ended. And that even though you love your husband, even though your baby is beyond anything you could have hoped for, you don't care about the fight, you can't engage.

There is a battle on for your mind and you can't lift a finger. You are stilted, stifled, stuck. You are standing on a magnet after eating a tonne of lead. You are drawn down. It is a physical sensation; you know it will only get stronger the more you try to stand up to it. You will buckle under its weight and split. You can't contain this situation, this disease, forever. Your mind isn't strong enough to hold it. For now, you can shut it down, you can walk away, you can keep your mouth shut and hope nothing falls out because naming it will be even worse.

But it is already bigger than you. You stand in the kitchen and wet yourself like a child. Something about the crying, either the force of it on your body, or the emotion, sets you off and you can't stop until you are done.

The realisation that you will have to confess to someone, somewhere, at some point, that this is bigger than you is too much to bear. You try to explain to your husband why you are suddenly terrified, shaking, crying. You hear yourself scraping at the surface, trying to unpick it for him, trying to help him understand. But all you can do is repeat again and again your fear that you will be taken away and locked in a ward, rubbed out and removed and left in the manner of all mad people, protesting your sanity as the doors close in on you sitting in your own filth.

As you say this, he holds you, tells you he won't let anyone steal you, he says he loves you and he doesn't hate you. He knows you've hardly slept for weeks and even though he hasn't either, that he will take charge tonight. He guides you to your bed and changes your clothes. As he wipes you down, he calls your socks 'booties'. It is a slip of the tongue, the language of fatherhood, nappies and newborns, mangling his own sleepy mind. But you wonder if he already suspects he is going to be taking care of all of you from now on.

Either way, the madness and the leakiness melt together; your body and your mind are dissolving. And even with an addled mind, you are starting to wonder: is being pissy the by-product or the cause of this disintegration?

Chapter 5

Six-week check

Due to my awful recovery, I don't make the first meet up with the other new mums from my class so I have the keen sense that I am already falling behind, missing out on the micro achievements of the early weeks, thanks to my stupid body and its slimy haemorrhages.

Thursday, late August 2007, coffee shop with eight mums and eight buggies crammed around a table creaking with breast pads

I look around the table at all the women from my antenatal group. We share the conspiratorial hush of witnesses to a crime, or jurors who have learned an unforgettable truth and can't unlearn it. We tell and re-tell our stories. Birth was a battlefield, and the aftermath a mad scramble and now the most prodded and examined amongst us, whose births were most mechanical or damaging, feel a bit like leftovers, like we've disappeared as people.

It's good, though, to know I wasn't the only one wrong-footed by the carnage, and though I'm slightly wired about returning to the scene of the crime for my six-week check, they chivvy me on. We're all new to this, they remind me, and the birth is finished now. It is time to enjoy our babies.

I look at mine. He looks happy enough, even though he will not keep his socks on no matter how many old ladies tell me off at bus stops. These women are kind though – we hardly know each other really but they tell me I am going to make a go of it, just get through my appointment and start moving forward.

I take a deep breath; maybe today will be the end of the medical madness and I can ride the wave of confidence the new mums have given me. Besides, because I am already on the cusp of madness, and to be fair to post-natal me, *desperately* trying to put a brave face on, I have planned plenty of activities for the day to displace any nagging doubts. Having forgotten the advice of our antenatal teacher that one thing a day is more than enough to do, and that we should prioritise recuperation in these early weeks, I've developed FOMO years before the phrase is popularised by social media.

Today's itinerary includes:

1 Meeting new mum friends for latte – DONE.
2 Getting my downstairs signed off by the consultant team – ON MY WAY.
3 Going to a baby cinema event –WHY NOT? And …
4 Driving down with my dad to the Isle of Wight. WHAT. A. DICK.

Within an hour, job two is in progress.

I sit in the pared-down appointment room, trying not to look at the barred windows, as a breezy female consultant runs through her list. I tell her, as I have told everyone so far, what's healing and what hurts, and she takes a peek and murmurs her approval at my very neat stitches.

I crack a little and cry quietly as I explain the last few weeks that brought me here, to the room with the complicated patients rather than to my friendly GP. I only stop crying when we talk mental health, and reassure us both with my horrified (truthful) response:

'No – of course I don't want to hurt my baby. He's *great*. None of this is his fault.'

I've admitted I'm still a little bit scared I might be getting depressed. The consultant looks up and gives me a moment even though she, like everyone else, wants to crack on with the August Bank Holiday.

'You've had a pretty difficult time you know, Luce,' she says kindly. 'I think anyone would be upset.'

But there's something about the neatness of the conversation that isn't quite right. Even if I avoid telling her about the waves of sadness, the flashbacks and the night-terrors, even if we ditch my suspicion I might have post-natal depression (PND), I think she hasn't 'got it'. Nobody's getting it: I really do feel very, very different 'down below'. She starts to talk about how it can take a while to feel normal, to heal, that I should be doing pelvic floor exercises.

'I'm trying ...' I start.

'I know it's hard to remember, but you'll really see a difference,' she continues, looking ruefully at my bulging file. 'It's useful to pick an activity you do regularly, in the morning, like loading the washing machine or washing up or doing your teeth, and do your exercises then.'

I stop. I close my eyes. My cheeks warm up.

I don't know what it is about this moment of silence. Maybe it reminds me of the delivery room that morning. Maybe it's the insight into the infernal fucking drudge of motherhood that means everyday activities are now stultifying housework rather than, I don't know, wanking or watching *Midsomer Murders*. Maybe it's the quiver of my son's breath as he sighs in his sleep, smelling me from a distance, hands like Beyoncé, face like a sleeping pope, or the milky circles appearing on my top. Or the catch of sunlight in my eye and pooling over my hospital notes. Or maybe I'm realising I'm (marginally) more fed up than I am tired. But suddenly I see my folly. I want to escape this place but I must get someone to hear the truth. I cannot cannot CANNOT listen to anymore standard advice that feels like it's for someone else.

'It isn't that. I do them every day but it's just ... even when I do, I can't really feel anything, not properly. When I squeeze, it's like ... a void.'

She cocks her head. Pen down. Swallowing a sigh to conceal her frustration at a patient chucking in a curveball just as she was about to send them away. Especially a patient whose gash she's already inspected.

'Tell me that again,' she says. 'How different does it feel?'

'Like it's broken. Like I can't work it. Sometimes I can't really tell at all that I'm weeing. I just start, or realise I am. And I don't know, I just feel like I'm wetting myself. A lot. But maybe I'm just tired. It's normal, isn't it?'

'Fuck,' I think, hearing myself and realising all at once that I might be one of *those* women who all the euphemisms and whispers were about as I was growing up. The whispers about Auntie this and Mrs So and So down the road that children aren't supposed to hear, faces pulled we aren't supposed to absorb, about the tribe of silent suffering women who'd had a baby and 'were never the same since'. Panic dawns and sets in in one breath, but my mouth is my most incontinent bit of all. I look away from her face and splurge it out:

'I just ... leak. If I laugh, or try to climb the stairs. Sometimes it just starts when I'm breastfeeding or holding the baby. I can't stop it. And nothing's in the right place anymore.'

'Pop back onto the bed,' she suggests. Less rakishly than I would have liked, but kindly. 'You aren't going to like this, but ...'

'Oh Christ!' I think. Frantic. She's going to say it is too big and buckety for her to put her fingers in, or that my poor little vag looks like a folded slice of salami because they've stitched it wrong, or that there's an abscess I've been too slovenly to spot, or more bloody placenta, and I'll be sent back to the labour ward. Or worse, worse than all that, that I'm pregnant again or there was another baby stuck up there all along.

It is even worse than that.

'I'd like you to cough for me,' she says. 'Nice big cough.'

I cringe. Until that point, I haven't really seen it as embarrassing, just strange. I've been so snow-blinded by all the medical trauma, and being a hulking slab of broken body pushed around a table, that I've forgotten how it feels to be a person, a social being, doing social things, normal things in front of other people. I realise I want to be protected. I can't cough: I will piss like a water fountain and it will make my stitches sting and my insides feel like they are about to topple out, only with no glorious compensation like a baby, just wee in a puddle on the table-bed. Also, it will probably go all over my thighs, and seep up behind my back onto my T-shirt, and I have to get to the cinema on a bus and I don't have anything spare to wear.

'I know you know what's going to happen, but don't hold back,' she says, firmly.

I half-cough and dribble.

'You can do better than that,' she says, encouragingly.

When she's looked, a lot, and I've spluttered from dripping to full gush, and she's (very gently) had a feel, she stands back, unsnaps her gloves and starts washing her hands.

'You have a prolapse,' she says with a sigh, her back to me for modesty's sake. I feel like I've disappointed her, though in retrospect, I think she just knew it was a crapshoot. And then it starts. Anatomical, diagnostic words invade the room. 'Severe' and 'stress incontinence', 'urgency' and 'voiding'. Questions about how many pads I use in a day and if I need them at night. Even in this avalanche, I sense sympathy seeping through her back. It makes me shudder.

'It feels like something's dropping down,' I offer.

She explains what a prolapse is: my uterus pushing into the wall of my vagina making a bulge. She explains it properly, and clearly, with medical terms.

I think, 'MY FUCKING WOMB IS FALLING OUT.'

'Does anything else make you leak?' she asks, as I clamber gracelessly down from the examination bed and let out another warm slick.

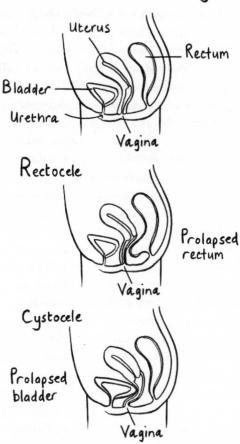

Normal Female Pelvic Anatomy

Uterus

Rectum

Bladder

Urethra

Vagina

Rectocele

Prolapsed
rectum

Vagina

Cystocele

Prolapsed
bladder

Vagina

And then I remember the worst thing. Somewhere in the murky world of attending classes, speaking to friends, asking tentative questions online, I'd got the idea we should have sex before the six-week check to make sure everything is working and report any problems. In reality, it isn't great advice, not least because everyone is individual and you and your doctors will know best, but at the time I wanted to be normal and do what I was supposed to. My husband is compliant by nature too. Both of us always the milk monitor. Always the narrator. And besides, the quick post-birth shag to make sure everything's fine had sounded like fun back when we were cracking jokes in the antenatal class and thought we'd covered all eventualities.

We did as we were told, of course. On the landing, in the half dark, with plenty of pillows and limited romance. Our bedroom dominated by the briefly sleeping infant. Should I tell her it happened then? Was that too much information, even for a doctor? Not for her to hear, necessarily – she talked about stretched and torn genitals all day long (what a job!) – but for me to tell?

I pull back the curtain to show myself completely. We lock eyes.

'Everything makes me wet myself,' says a tinny, defiant voice.

She nods, to indicate compassion is appropriate but that she can't give it. Neither of us has time for me to start crying again. It might never end. She picks up her pen and proposes a plan.

'You'll need to see the physiotherapists here immediately,' she says. 'I'll make the referral now.'

I look aghast: I can't come back here. I can't. It will feel like death or torture. I'll hyperventilate in the lobby.

'There are all sorts of things they can do these days. Don't worry. Honestly,' she says, thinking, probably, that I'm afraid of indignity.

'It's not that. I …'

'They have classes in the gym …'

THEY HAVE CLASSES? IN A GYM? All of us pissing together and not getting picked in PE? My anxiety is at fever pitch. I'm an incontinent *and* I have to go back to fucking gym class?

'… but I think you probably need to see someone one to one.'

Is that better?

My baby squawks. I see his toes peeping out from his yellow blanket. Simple. Edible. Mine.

I almost smile. I'm brave. I can do it for him, for us. I can at least try.

'They really are very good here.'

I close my eyes, but I feel her look through my lids. I realise she's reassessing the degree of my upset.

'I think you might need some trauma counselling too,' she adds, snatching an additional referral sheet for my file.

You think?

That day, when I realised I went beyond the occasional 'oops moment', remained seared on my memory. A year later I wrote to a friend:

> *'I think the Isle of Wight will probably be nice but I feel a bit antsy about it because – and I know this is really stupid – it is exactly what we did last year and that Thursday was one of the grimmest days of my life.'*

But I'm not sure this is surprising. Diagnosis is a bummer, even if you know it is coming, even if you've been honest enough with yourself to know something is probably wrong.

Thursday, late August 2007, on the way to baby cinema, and then a road trip

As we, my son and I, wait for the massive and creaking hospital lifts I feel robbed of something. Punished for my honesty. Womanning up has just earned me bonus humiliation. Physio. And trauma counselling.

After three sets of stairs and with my womb hanging somewhere near my ankles, I get to baby cinema and watch *The Bourne Ultimatum*. I cry when Paddy Considine is shot and get over-invested in Jason Bourne's lack of backstory. But my baby loves the light and shadows, and cracks one of his first proper smiles as

Matt Damon kicks the shit out of someone. Perhaps it is as cathartic for him as it is for me.

I look over at the attractive and neat-looking younger mums in the cinema; in my sticky T-shirt (milk) and bottoms (wee), I feel lacking. I realise later they are nannies though. A different tribe. 'They probably brushed their teeth this morning,' I think caustically. *Those were the fucking days*.

And then we start our Isle of Wight road trip: three hours driving, a ferry and a chain ferry for extra measure. Easy. I still cannot believe I did it. My father collects me and the baby from home and we ride in the back of his car. The baby starts crying. He only stops when we hit 70mph or more. This makes the hour of standstill roadworks in West London an Ealing comedy rip-off of *Speed*, only I don't get to kiss Keanu or Sandra Bullock and instead half-garrotte myself in the seatbelt and straps trying to breastfeed my son from above his car seat as he explodes with rage.

My chaotic early weeks of motherhood are complete when we literally miss the boat, hearing the clang of the gates as we pull in to a Southampton car park and see the great ship heave its way over the Solent. My dad does something kind. He gets me a foot passenger ticket for another ferry and arranges for Mum to meet us and cuddle us on the other side, while he waits for the next crossing. The water is black and solid in the night air. But it has the memory of summer glow, the shimmer of late night seaside, when the sand's still warm, still fresh from sunbathers early in the day. It lacks the bite of winter. But it is large and expansive and shiny enough to soothe me.

I reflect on the day, grasping onto the doctor's initial assessment that bad shit has happened and I'm probably not depressed, having immediately forgotten her trauma remark. I'm very tired. My mum feeds me hot crab. But I've done too much clambering and running around to make good conversation, too much talking and leaking and remembering, too much swirling fear tipping me off balance like a spongey headache.

It is a significant weekend. I experience unparalleled joy, crack my first fucked-up fanny joke, and start to lose my mind. And I thought my original to-do list was ambitious.

I see the pleasure other people get from my baby. It is the best bit of motherhood that people forget to tell you, all those insights into love. A family friend describes my son as 'adorabubble', setting off fireworks in my fallopian tubes. My dad leans in and kisses his head, and I see the love, all the love that he ever had for me, for my sisters, from his family, that he built with my mum. The past and future of love in the pad of one little kiss.

My first foray into fanny humour comes the next morning. The joke about my broken foof is much like the first poo post-delivery. It hurts me more than I thought it would, and possibly causes further damage. Also, it stinks and it isn't very funny.

Instinctively, we turn to humour as a defence. I am very defensive. I am sitting in a beautiful garden that mines the microclimate for all of nature's verdant glory. It's behind a plain Victorian house but combines fig trees and tomatoes, statues and bonsai, has a lush overgrown meadow patch and spikey bursts of green and purple spilling out through the rockeries. Flowers billow in the breeze, scents dancing in the air. It's a garden built from warmth, in a house that thrills with the hope and expectation that there will be friends, and children, and last-minute guests. The cutlery and plates don't match, the strength and kindness is uniform and all-welcoming.

So it wasn't very fair, really, that a family friend (who also knew me from babyhood) should say the line 'tear you a new arsehole' in a conversation on *the other side of the garden*, to *somebody else*, and I should interject, loud and spiky:

'Enough already – some of us have actually torn themselves a new arsehole. And it hasn't even healed yet.'

It was a start.

I think I knew then that humour would be a blight and a saviour, but I sank into familial love as the day played out and didn't consider how casually I had just set myself up as the butt of the joke. A stinky scapegoat for everything. Or spot how much I'd started saying crude things about my body, out loud, to reflect my shock and outrage. And I certainly didn't realise that perhaps you don't need to do any of that at all, because most people, most, are kind enough to listen, share that shock and be kind, if you are really, really upset. You don't *need* to swear and shout about it.

Even at my saddest, I am eternally romantic though, so when I watch the sun set I just think, 'It's all going to be all right, isn't it?'

I embrace the good as hard as I can. There is a baby. And summer. And, finally, an ice cream. My son is the very hungry caterpillar, pink-faced in a green playsuit. A curious Victorian bather in the shade. I can still see beauty in the world.

The next morning I breastfeed on a terrace by the sea wall in the blue glow of the just-dawn light; the world is sleeping but the sea is alive and persistent.

The fresh clean air reminds me of Sylvia Plath and her poem 'Morning Song' where she's 'cow-heavy' in her floral nightie, bewitched by her baby's 'handful of notes', that 'rise like balloons'. Sylvia's clear that love set him going 'like a fat gold watch'. I muse on Plath for a few seconds but she feels too portentous a reference and I push her back into my head.

I also learn practical skills that weekend, like how to spot open arms that might hold your baby for half an hour when you think you might die from being tired.

But mostly, I dissolve. Deep down, especially as I enter the sea, tits hard and hot with milk. I sting, but I know it isn't the vicious salt that's the problem. I can see the Spinnaker Tower looming on the mainland just across from the beach. The little channel is too small. There isn't enough expanse to hide me. I want the sea to be spreading and engulfing, not a water highway with parameters. When we get back to my parents' place, I find myself following my baby's sounds through the house like a song, drifting through my own mind as I stumble around. I know something's up.

When I'm researching this book, I go back through my emails and drafts and find one of the few things I did write on my maternity leave:

You are lying on the floor in your parents' house and it skims against you. You think, 'I could just lie down under the waves.'

Your arms and shoulders are heavy before the thought has finished. Your knees ache. It isn't a suicidal thought. It isn't a plan. It isn't fully formed. But it is real, and it hangs in the air.

You know you wouldn't go and drown yourself. You wouldn't jump off the sea wall. You wouldn't fling yourself from the ferry. But when you stand still, you can't fight the feeling that you might.

A switch in your gut flicks. Somewhere inside you, you already kind of know you will never forget it. You walk over to your baby who is lying on the floor and lie down next to him.

Macy Gray is singing 'I Try' on your father's stereo. You think about the song, you gaze at your perfect baby, you relax. Your sense of dis-ease begins to dissolve. You think that maybe, just maybe, the song, the moment, your love for your son, has saved you. You look at your baby. He is more beautiful and perfect than you ever thought possible. He transcends your imagination. You think this is the end. But this thought was just the beginning.

I often think of her, that new mum me, swirling in the aftershock, floating towards the darkness, and how sorry I am she didn't know how to say it all.

I want to hold her and stroke her hair, because she was right to be afraid. It *was* just the beginning.

Chapter 6

Damage assessment

The biggest revelations of my maternity leave didn't come to me in a doctor's office or a physio suite. They hit me in my own living room, as I was hiding from the world, crying on the sofa during *Countdown*.

October 2007, afternoon, watching Channel 4 in a lounge strewn with nappies and hospital letters

Dr Phil Hammond is in Dictionary Corner, sitting next to national treasure Susie Dent, the woman who holds the whole show together by finding long words no one has heard of, and understanding grammar. Hammond is a medic, comedian and author, nicknamed 'Doctor Phil'. Usually, I can give him a run for his money if I play along at home, though today he's panning me.

In fact, I'm wondering if 'baby brain' is a real thing, rather than a sexist myth, when, suddenly, an eight-letter word emerges from the jumble of vowels and consonants and springs into my mind. PERINEAL. Boom.

I scribble down my triumph bitterly, trying not to wake the baby. At least my experience means I can spell that one.

Doctor Phil spots it too. Of course he does. And then quips that most women don't know where their perineum is until they have a baby. The audience laughs, as Des O'Connor side-eyes the original number witch Carol Vorderman. Susie and I just grimace.

Susie, because whenever anyone says a word she has to stare at the definition on her laptop, and in this case, it presumably reads '*relating to the area between the anus and the scrotum or vulva.*'

And me, because Doctor Phil has just described my intimate illiteracy on the actual telly. I'm taking it personally that I'm such an easy target. And worst of all, I can't clamber on to my feminist soap box and screech about the patriarchy because he's bloody well right too. Where exactly is (or was?) my perineum? Had I ever really known?

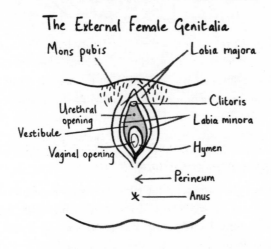

The External Female Genitalia

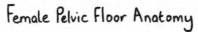

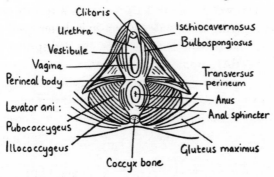

Female Pelvic Floor Anatomy

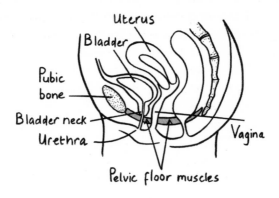

Female Pelvic Muscles

Labels: Uterus, Bladder, Pubic bone, Bladder neck, Urethra, Vagina, Pelvic floor muscles

I'd definitely *heard* of it before. And while there may have been some ghastly discussion of massaging it in antenatal class, I'd powered down to amber by then, out of terror and disgust. And as for my pelvic floor? I was in regular treatment to fix it, but did I even know what it looked like?

And what else was missing from my sex education (which I realise, as I try to recall it, is a crazed collage of thoughts and images from an eclectic range of sources)? Soap operas, books, magazines, friends, torturous lessons with embarrassed biology teachers, and hormonal boys staring at a diagram in which the womb looks eerily like an angry ram.

I definitely learned about periods and pregnancy along the way, but I only skirted the physiological and hormonal foundations, the things that leave women like me sitting on a towel to protect the sofa.

Spring 1988, school coach, windy country lane near Loughborough, on the way to swimming

I like swimming because we don't have to change with the boys. For normal PE we all change together in our classroom, and everyone can see your pants and vest and chickenpox scars.

Of the five girls in my year, one is already wearing a bra, and we think one of the third years might already need one too. My mum has offered me a delicate denim look crop top for mine, even though they only quiver a tiny bit when I shake them. Also, I have *hairs*.

This means puberty is coming. Puberty means spots, boyfriends, the fourth-year trip and French kissing. I think it also means I can have babies.

I know a lot about babies, because my mum is having twins. I've been on a hospital tour and demo-ed a birthing chair when none of the women wanted a go. And I've got a book that shows a foetus as she grows. She has an alien face and see-through fingers. Babies inside their mummies look like E.T.

I am ready for womanhood and have stopped sticking cushions up my jumper to play at being pregnant. I know where tummy buttons come from and why they look like the knot on a party balloon. I think Umbilical sounds like a Womble.

I am a bit hazy on where exactly I keep my eggs but today will change all that.

My friend's big sister has given her a leaflet that she sent off for from *Jackie*. I'm so jealous my eyes stretch wide.

This is the most wicked thing that has ever happened in our boring bit of the East Midlands. Ever. We pass it around the back seat all the way to swimming and back.

Published by Tampax, it has pastel coloured cartoons of fannies with labels. It is brilliant. The perineum isn't one of the highlights.

It gives details about flow, heavy and light, shows our ovaries, like boiled sweets, and our tube, called a 'vagina'. The tube is key. It is where a tampon fits. The leaflet tells us Tampax tampons absorb the mess. I can't imagine mine with a string hanging out.

We memorise the words. New ones like 'ovary', 'menstrual' and 'applicator', and new meanings of old words like 'towel', 'monthly' and 'on'. I feel closer to being a teenager than ever before.

We learn about spotting, starting and the 28 days. We marvel at the science. Even the warning of cramps doesn't dampen our anticipation. The leaflet doesn't talk about flooding, or egg white cervical mucus, or the leap of faith of getting a tampon high enough up. But that doesn't matter. It is clear the universe is inviting us into a secret club. We are at the start of something big.

My introduction to sex and reproduction was analogue; I learned about my anatomy by secretly reading my mother's feminist bookshelf. Too early for the Internet, I topped up with school, gossip, and glossy magazines, and I only learned the rudest words aged 26, reading the call girl blog *Belle de Jour*.

The best book my mum had was *Our Bodies, Ourselves*, an outsized hardback standing proud with *The Female Eunuch*, *The Women's Room*, *Jane Fonda's Workout Book* and something by British childbirth activist and author Sheila Kitzinger (unfortunately for me, not her 1971 classic *Giving Birth: How It Really Feels*).

My mum's *Our Bodies, Ourselves* had been around all my life. A group of women wrote it together. Its success was in combining collective female experience with straight-talking medical information. It felt quaint by the '90s, though now it feels like the blueprint for today's surge of female empowerment, from demystifying menstrual blood on social media to putting suffragette statues in Parliament Square.

As a teen, I would spend hours when no one else was home, lying on the dining room floor staring at the diagrams and drawings and actual photos of everything. Unashamed pubes curling proudly between women's legs and line drawings of breasts. There were thorough medical descriptions of childbirth too, and babies' screaming faces wearing their mother's leg-tops as a hat, but I didn't dwell on how that might feel or how much effort it would be or how big a 10 cm circle actually was.

I marvelled at it all, though I thought it was going a bit far when they suggested using a mirror to look at my cervix. The angles were unthinkable.

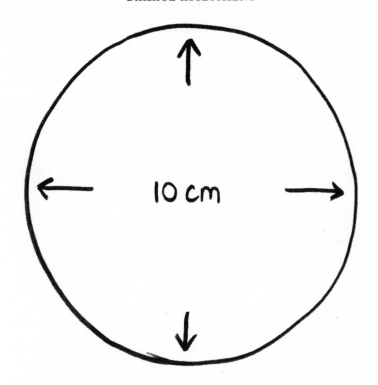

The first time I even considered looking anywhere near my cervix was at 9 a.m. the day after I went into labour, when the midwife Kay offered me a mirror to see my son's head crowning. But the risk of looking at my fanny at that point, even if I could have stopped shaking, did not seem worth it. I tried to quip that the time for admiring it was long gone but I was too slurry and my husband had to translate and say, 'SHE DOESN'T WANT TO LOOK.'

Even high on pethidine and trauma, oozing and performing, I knew. I knew I was broken and that it wasn't just the midwives who would have their work cut out putting me back together again. What I didn't know was how anyone would ever be able to assess the damage if no one knew what it looked like in the first place.

1989–91 secondary school playgrounds, various

My friends and I now give each other daily updates on what is happening in our knickers. If we've started our periods or might be about to, what signs are there in our sticky gussets.

We are at secondary school and we've all sent off to the tampon company now; we have matching pink plastic holders to hide our samples. Discretion is the order of the day throughout my tweens and teens. The sanitary products industry is on a marketing kick to ensure no one will ever know, or be able to tell, when we finally start.

Lil-Lets even has its branding printed on clear wrapping. Look, you tear it off and the writing disappears. You just have a small blue box. It could be anything. *Anything.*

It is something secret for girls to know. And although it contradicts our real desire, which is to talk with fascination about blobs and pink strings and leaking day and night, we've walked eyes open into an absurd and dangerous pact. We women, and girls, will shut up and put up with all the bodily grot and not make a fuss about any of it in case it gets embarrassing for the boys. We will pay VAT on tampons unthinkingly, and embrace a silence that affects everyone.

As we hit the 1990s I get obsessed with feminism because I'm perturbed at the contradictions in the new wave of empowerment. '*Whooah Bodyform*' is a standard put-down for anyone in a strop, but all the girls laugh when our PSD (personal and social development) teacher tells us a girl in her previous school thought the sticky bits of pads attached to your labia rather than your pants. I think, 'We are not all shaped for confidence.'

I still hadn't ever seen a Tena Lady box or heard of continence pads. The Bodyform adverts were causing enough ripples. But the denial wasn't mine. Incontinence *was* hushed-up back then. Bizarre but true – market researchers launching continence pads in the UK in the 1980s had to inform the local police in advance when they went to do door-to-door research, in case housewives and old ladies dialled 999 at the mere mention of such a taboo-laden product. Even now, discussing continence aids is an area seen by market researchers as one shrouded in taboo – a sector where caution and sensitivity are needed and where finding a large sample may be hard – though a late 2010s push for awareness might be shifting that view.

When my sex education lesson gets down to it with a module called 'Growth' we fill in the Latin words on a diagram of reproductive organs and try to ignore the giggling that dominates: the gagging sounds from the back of the lab every time the teacher says vagina, the salacious lip-licking and sound effects at any hint of genitals on the overhead projector.

I call the boys in our class 'sexist', but there's no especial desire from anyone to do anything other than look stern. They call me 'Maggie Thatcher' in reply.

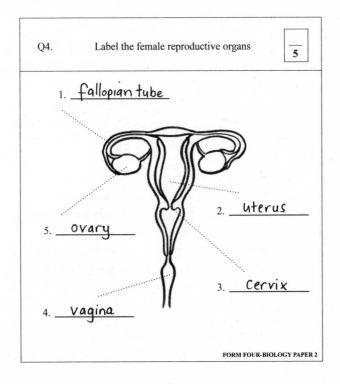

Q4.   Label the female reproductive organs   5

1. fallopian tube

2. uterus

3. cervix

5. ovary

4. vagina

FORM FOUR-BIOLOGY PAPER 2

'Fuck you!' I think, and hurl the most below-the-belt insult I have back over my shoulder: 'Which one of you fainted during the giving birth video again?'

I use the tampon information leaflet as ironic 'recycled wrapping paper' for my best friend's fifteenth birthday present amidst blushes and giggles, before we get back to learning about actual sex from *More* magazine's 'position of the fortnight', agog at the angles and sliced-in-half pictures that show how a penis shaft fits snugly into a vagina in so many different arrangements. Pop stars say to exercise our bits by stopping our pee to make us better at sex, and we spot vulvas echoed everywhere: in Georgia O'Keefe's flower paintings, the swoop of the Scottish Widow's black hood and Edvard Munch's 'The Scream' with his big fanny mouth.

For me, at 15, this feels evolved enough.

When I think back over the past, on the sofa, with my baby, I realise the professionals working on helping me improve my continence have changed-up the script I learned at school. Early incontinence is a far weirder gear shift than becoming a menstruator. Immediately, they point out that the two systems – gastro and reproduction – are not as separate as I'd always thought. I hear words I don't know or have no proper definition for, words that I don't remember from any textbook. 'Anterior prolapse', 'uterine', 'os' and 'rectocele' for a start. *Sexy.*

Worse, they keep yakking on about my bladder and urethra, my bowels and anus and my sphincters. Yes, plural – there are loads (two up your bum for a start!). I've heard these words, of course, but I had only thought of them as separate from my reproductive system. Waste disposal units in a neighbouring locale, not potential collateral damage.

These people, who I now see more than my friends and family, these nurses, doctors, physiotherapists, are throwing new knowledge at me. Informing me that, like sphincters, there are many kinds of incontinence. It isn't as simple as a little bit of wee coming out when you laugh.

Stress urinary incontinence (SUI) is the most common and I definitely have that. The stress isn't about being furious, it's about leaking caused by physical stress or exertion. But there's also urge, mixed, functional, double.

They give me homework. My physio even brings down the dusty plastic model pelvis from her office shelves to show me in 3D where my muscles aren't working. She's re-mapping the landscape of my nether regions as a precarious war zone, rather than the fountain of new life and womanhood. I feel like an absolute chump.

It turns out, by the way, that *Our Bodies, Ourselves* does have a section on pelvic floor muscles and exercises, but as a teen I never got that far as it was in the back, with diseases of ageing and decrepitude, like arthritis. Something of *Our Bodies, Ourselves* stays with me though, and from the start of my first pregnancy I seek out collective female voices. For me this means logging on to Internet mum forums. I think it will just be prams chat and due date countdowns, but it turns out the place comes into its own when I need to find solace for my broken fanny.

October 2007, evening, lounge strewn with nappies, hospital letters, sitting in front of a laptop with an open bottle of wine

A special clique of birth injury survivors has readily taken me under their wing, giving me a crew of surrogate big sisters, each with their own knackered-nethers story, cheering me on when I admit I need fanny physio.

There's an unwritten hierarchy of terrible birth experiences, of course. I'm on the team, but not a star player, thank Christ. My tear is second degree, we're both alive, and I don't have an ostomy bag. But these women understand why I sometimes don't feel lucky. We don't talk about our intimate brokenness *all* the time, but we do delight in damage comparison when it comes up.

In tonight's outlandish thread they are using sharp adjectives to talk stitches. Standard. 'I have material for *that*,' I think. My contributions go something like this:

'Everyone who sees my scars and my stitches says they're beautiful,' (set-up). 'The midwives on the home team actually name-checked the lady who stitched me up. They were purring over her handiwork *before* they looked at my notes … (wait for it) … I'm beginning to wonder if she embroidered her signature on my snatch.' (Boom!)

The post explodes with PMSL emojis. Another poster asks what it looks like now and I confess I don't dare check.

My best guess is 'Mr Twit's beard', so I'm glad we're anonymous.

'Is the little man still in his canoe?' she counters. Bold.

I hoot and as I've had a glass of wine since my husband came home, think 'Damn it, I can do this.' I go to have a look now the swelling has gone down. There are considerably more frills and lines, but yes, he bloody well is still there.

'Just about!' I reply in triumph. We fill the screen with weeping smileys.

The laughing and the looking has touched a damaged nerve though: we might have broken through the anatomical taboo, but nobody's talking about the emotional side.

'I feel quite shit about it all and how much it's taken away from me emotionally,' I confess. The thread falls silent. There's kindness, but no mirroring for my gloomy thoughts. Even there, in the clit-nit-picking autopsy, the despair is muted.

Canoe woman eventually comes back and says she can't really talk about how it makes her feel. This is the problem when two taboos start co-sleeping.

Part Two

AFTERMATH –
WHO AM I NOW?

Chapter 7

Depression

Loads of research shows links between depression and incontinence. The stats vary depending on the type of study, but not much. I know this from one of my middle-of-the-night Google health searches, looking for help with sore skin. Depression is right up there with other problems that are linked to incontinence and probably made worse by these complications too. It's a stark list: social isolation, sleep deprivation (from getting up for a wee), UTIs (urinary tract infections), fractures (from falls dashing for a wee, a huge problem with geriatric patients), chafing and urine burns.

Despite all the evidence about incontinence demolishing what doctor's term patients' 'quality of life', for years no professional I see makes explicit to me the link between my depression and my leaking. This makes it easy for me, the patient, to blame myself when I end up on antidepressants. It makes my lackings – of knowledge, resourcefulness, muscle strength and resilience – feel like the reason I've succumbed to feeling so sad.

Interestingly, when I have some time and distance, I find that there is an increasingly strong body of research pointing out not just that incontinence sucks, but also that it can be a specific key predictor in the likelihood of post-natal depression. Women with incontinence are, in fact, *almost twice as likely to develop PND*. It truly is a condition that keeps on giving. Published in Canada in 2011, one study showed the five strongest predictors of depression after childbirth were urinary incontinence; the mother being under 25; readmissions to hospital; breastfeeding not working; and self-reported health issues to do with birth.

I didn't quite have a clean sweep with my first. I was over 25, and had lucky tits, but the rest though? You've read it.

The study said incontinence was a surprise entry as previously it had received little attention in research (good old taboos) and noted that, scientifically speaking, the research community did not yet 'fully understand the reasons incontinence is linked to depression'. I toy with ringing them up to explain the lethal pairing of total stigma and being told it is normal, so that feeling crazy for hating it plays a big part, along with, I suspect, the cost of continence aids and the way pissing yourself all the time precludes getting on with normal day-to-day life, let alone joyous things, like laughing.

But I don't know this at the time, so bad thoughts start clogging my brain.

'I must have bottled my own hang-ups and hysterics and saved them up as an explosive canister to chuck at the flames of distress when I had this baby,' I think. 'This is my own doing. I'm being punished for my over-confidence and now everyone will know I am bad underneath (and stupid).'

Incontinence and birth trauma are such social, psychological, and sexual disasters that I feel erased, somehow. They also make me feel like a fool, especially on good days when I don't have an accident, or we get something right, like a family trip to the zoo, and I think, 'Jesus, I've made the whole thing up.'

Part of that is the admonishing silence. My pissy knickers are not my fault, but it is too embarrassing to talk about them. It doesn't matter that my broken body shouldn't be shameful, or that I haven't committed a crime, incontinence has the same effect. You can't talk about it if you are polite; it's too dirty, too undignified.

By adding depression and trauma into the mix, my story started to splinter and deteriorate, and became impossible to follow or unpick, even as I was living it. The days and nights and memories collided and ran in parallel. Terrible months, when my depression raged, were still punctuated by sweetness and explosions of love for my son, whose insistent momentum – growing, changing, developing, reaching out and past me day-by-day, forging his own path and personality – dragged me along with him.

The monotony and sluggishness of my physio 'improvements' and the rapid-fire madness of my broken mind roamed wildly, as I got myself up, returned to work, fought for a social life and started all over again each day.

I started to have three parallel ways of expressing and understanding myself:

1   Leaky Luce is sad. She offers brittle shows of resilience and ploughs on towards help, buoyed by disbelief, shock and compliance. She's quite intense, I suspect, but mostly I feel sorry for her. She's trying to sort out something nearly impossible, while exhausted and in shock, and she's giving it her best shot.

2   Mad Luce sees herself through the critical voice of a God-like narrator that takes over her mind *in the second person* when nice Leaky Luce isn't strong enough to tell her to shut the fuck up, and boy, does she cut like a knife. She also, I realise, barely accepts that spending so much time with a chafed crotch and in the weird submission of medical appointments has any bearing on her state of mind, or ability to learn parenting. She doesn't wonder why other people aren't hyperventilating outside the doctor's surgery, she just assumes Leaky Luce is an idiot and a drama queen. She's

the worse sort of forthright too: a bitter, angry, judgemental juggernaut.

3 There is another me too – Mum Luce. Mainly she is always late.

I start writing things down as my mind divides. These memories are hard to grasp even now when I can cross-check them with letters and emails. It seems I was striving fruitlessly to unite the different strands of me, peppering my record with snatches of insight that I clung to, to make sense of myself.

For example, my A-Level English teacher taught me the E.M. Forster quote 'Only connect!' when I was 16. I wrote it down then because I was pretentious, not having read any of his books. But I write it all over my notebooks when I get depressed. When I look it up, and read it in context, in his novel *Howards End* it reads like a prophetic roadmap to getting better. A commandment against living life in fragments:

> *'Only connect! That was the whole of her sermon. Only connect the prose and the passion, and both will be exalted, and human love will be seen at its height. Live in fragments no longer.'*

It feels so wise. Right up with the last line of *Some Like It Hot*. Maybe back then, somewhere inside me, I know it: words and stories will save me in the end.

I keep a bastardised version of the *Some Like It Hot* quote scribbled in my notebook too, as a future weapon, to defuse the embarrassment when I make a mess or my body doesn't improve. Even then, I know it has potential, a perfect punchline for my fleshy disgrace: 'No body's perfect,' I'll say, with a wink.

Thinking too much about my mind is like drinking a cocktail laced with arsenic. One part thought crystallisation: rational, useful, and hopeful. And three parts open fucking door for my critical mania to really hit her stride. This diary excerpt says it all.

October 2007, Scruffy GP surgery, London

You have never been mad. You have never been 'mental'. Hysterical – perhaps. Manic – yes. OTT, a lousy drunk, very upset, shocked, shocking, sweary, dramatic, angry – all those things. But never, you know, really unstable. Not as an adult at least. Never one of the people everyone, strangers even, actually worry about doing something dreadful. And never diagnosed with anything that you could look up in a textbook.

And yet, despite spending a whole night panicking you were going to jump out of your rotting sash window, when you found yourself, propelled by your husband's dread and fear, sitting in your doctor's surgery in a pair of pyjamas, you were still expecting that she wouldn't believe you. That she would send you away. That she'd accept your front and say really, you were okay, making a fuss, even, to be crying all the time.

She might be sorry that you've had a rough week or two, pushing out blood clots and thinking you were going to die, but she would hardly care that you were starting to seriously believe everything in the world was going wonky.

You truly thought that she would tell you to 'pull yourself together'. Like the midwife who shouted, 'Compose yourself, Mrs Brett' when you were screaming. When you were too pussy to shout back, 'MRS Brett is my mother. You aren't even using my NAME.'

In your head, the script for this meeting was already written. But your doctor hasn't read the script. She doesn't send you away. She listens. She notes down your terrible thoughts, and before you've even come close to the worst bits, while you are still skirting round the outsides, saying, 'I think I'm probably sounding crazy and not making any sense …', she interrupts with, 'Well, I think you are depressed.'

She gives you a questionnaire. You laugh, bitterly, at the trite phrases about hurting yourself, no hope for the future, and the range of options it offers – not at all, some days, more than half the days, nearly every day. But before you know it, you are skipping down the page like you've forgotten the context is you, even as you think it is a waste of time: Who would tell the truth? How can these bland slices of melo-drama, these 'options', say anything about you? They feel like the questions in women's magazine quizzes or customer surveys. Even then, you're racing down the sheet ticking 'every day' for nearly everything.

You realise later you could tell the truth then, not because you weren't ashamed or horrified of the simple answers or the rage and terror beneath them, but because you have already started to think about how you could tell it as a funny story if you ever admit any of this has happened ...

'Do you want to kill yourself? Which half of the days?' HA HA HA HA HA.

You hand it back and she adds up your score. You are back at the top of the class: severely depressed. Simultaneously, you both notice you haven't filled in one of the questions, the one about concentration.

HA HA HA HA HA. More bleak humour for your sitcom life. She prescribes some medicine but you still think it is probably out of pity.

So you plough on, regardless. You don't take your tablets, or tell your mother, or admit to anyone else that you've let them all down, you don't even log back on to your mums' forum and admit they were right when they suggested the GP.

You arrive late at another meet up with the lovely, normal women you met in your classes, the women you giggled with about baby names. Over coffee, you forget yourself and say that during the birth you thought you were going to die. Reveal, in fact, that you hoped you were going to die.

One of the mums looks stricken.

'Oh, Luce, you didn't really think that, did you?' she says, because she's really, really nice.

But you can't take her kindness when you are so wanting. You bluster on and hope they don't remember it, but you've caught a whiff of the distance between you and all the other mothers. They are drinking decaf coffee but you are back in the delivery room, wondering when in the mess of the last few hours you removed your pants and put on this flowery gown. In the butcher's shop, the too-bright lights, with the worried faces and the great big clock. Images flash: a gloved hand, blood-soaked bed socks, people dressed in blue staring at your fanny as you push yourself so hard you think you'll fly backwards.

No one thing that happened to you was horrid enough to be 'really' traumatic. Even compared to the stories around this table. Nobody did die. People keep reminding you this is all that matters. You should be grateful. (You are.) Your labour produced a lovely boy. (You know.) And yet ...

To avoid spiralling down, you say something outlandish about getting fisted by a doctor and throw in a true story about looking up to see three student midwives, like a spray of angels, talking about your 'repair' and one of them asking, with genuine curiosity, 'Does that bit go with that bit?'

Back on track, Brett. Everybody shrieks. It is only just over the boundaries of being nice. You hope no one is laughing too nervously.

And then it happens. Days, weeks, moments later? You can't tell. But you are back in a doctor's surgery, dressed this time. You hear a woman talking half to herself, softly but insistently, and half to the female GP and the (horrified-looking) medical student learning about family practice, sitting beside her.

The woman says she has given up. She feels like she is in a battle she can't win. She doesn't have the will to fight. She's falling backwards, submerging, time has dissolved. Throughout her constant quiet chatter, she keeps kissing her baby and her eyes weep insistently, persistently, as if with a momentum of their own. She says she hates herself, she explains she is a failure. She rationalises, she is brutal, she is persuasive as she talks in paragraphs, punctuated with things that sound like they are supposed to be jokes. She hates herself, and she is worthless. She doesn't want to hurt herself. But she isn't sure she won't. She doesn't 'want' to kill herself, she just wants things to stop. For events to slow down, instead of cascading and firing off around her.

She says she feels that she isn't real any more, like she has started to disappear. Like she is watching herself in a movie. Her life plays out as she is stuck in time, a voyeur of her own thoughts. She's frightened and frightening, her eyes shine too hard, her voice reverberates off her teeth like she's whispering into a tin. Her hair, her dancing hands, her costume, her baby – they all look faintly familiar.

And then, shit, you realise the truth. You know that woman: that woman is you.

When I tried to record that first two years of being mad at the time, my thoughts were punitive, relying on my instability, my fear and my distress to suggest an inability to quite hang onto reality. In my dark moments I searched for the comic in a showcase of horror that I hid beneath the upbeat Facebook shares. Mostly, though, I was on a mental health rollercoaster.

People I have never met read my questionnaire score and thrust therapists, theories, and labels upon me. I meet a START team, mental health nurses, and a counsellor who describes the post-birth body as a 'gutted fireplace'. These multiple voices speculating about my mind add to my growing sense that maybe I'm not real anymore. My thoughts can't be interpreted neatly. A psychotherapist I meet later patiently points out that PTSD symptoms include 'dissociation'. For me, this means watching my life as a boring play, forced into withdrawal as I become my own critical audience.

I see a proper psychiatrist, a busy Polish doctor who I meet in a tacky-floored side room of a building devoid of décor. My husband sits outside, jiggling the boy and worrying. She delivers the good news that I am not nearly ill enough to stay in hospital but makes some suggestions about mood-controlling drugs. She also asks if I can afford private counselling, given the waiting lists. I agree to pursue it. The trauma counselling was only a few sessions, it couldn't jumpstart me out of my state, so I bumble between private and NHS therapists for months.

But dipping in and out of therapeutic chit-chat sends your internal barometer screwy, especially the bit of your gut that lets you know if what you are saying is terrifying to others. I struggle to remember what constitutes non-mad behaviour around normals. Like when I let slip to Cat one day that in the peaks of my desperation, as our boys rolled around on her Ikea rug, I had been tempted to jump off her balcony. I drop it in like nothing and, not noticing her response to this blithe admission, add that I talked myself out of it by thinking it would have been so terrible for her to see that mess, and how it might have affected her flat price, and how she would have had to tell her baby (or mine) about it one day.

'Also, you are my friend,' she points out, gently, sanely. 'It would have been awful because you are my friend.'

The drama of mental healthcare is difficult but so is the tedium. The long waiting lists are hard. But so is the telling and retelling of your most shameful and upsetting thoughts, and the weirdness of taking yourself to the brink, and then being told 'time's up', 'one more session to go', 'see you next week'.

Depression is also difficult to manage when people expect you still to be on cloud nine about having a perfect new baby, never mind that a fear of leaking means your mind is splitting. A part of me *was* a bouncy enthusiastic new mum, another this increasingly institutionalised outpatient, losing my marbles and my bladder control. I was bamboozled by the contradictions, but also the startling truth of that time: I still needed to get up in the morning. Even if I couldn't. Even if I felt wrecked. Even when I was wretched. But also, I still wanted to, for him: my boy, my driver. Mania and action almost always triumphing over full submersion.

Chapter 8

Survival

Out of the tatters of the first broken weeks and months I emerged, no victorious all-conquering yummy mummy, but a lumpy, yukky me, soaked in her own wee. Sad and mad I may have been, but I was still alive enough to know that life was marching on and I had to develop some coping strategies. Ways to find myself in the mayhem and, if not, reach a peak of actualisation, at least carve a life in Tena Lady so I could taste some of the glory in teaching my son to wave at the baby in the mirror with his plump starfish hands. And if tramping around town with a two-tonne buggy in tow taught me anything, it was that coping with incontinence is more than just finding the right size and shape of pads. To avoid the dishonour of a wet patch you need a uniform.

As summer cracked into autumn 2007 I realised that I'd be back at work in a few months; if I didn't solve the dressing problem, I'd get marooned watching *Grey's Anatomy* and crying all day and my life would never carry on. I needed clothes that would hide my multitude of stains and sins, and let me escape. Clothes that could skim over pad bulges, and wouldn't chafe or make the pads rustle. Clothes good enough to withstand multiple washes, or cheap enough to replace, and that could be folded and hidden under a buggy. I went for expediency and length: long cardigans, long tunics and dresses over leggings. All, for style and practicality, in black.

For the worst times, thankfully infrequent, I needed to get over myself and use proper disposable pants (adult nappies). Despite being more expensive than saffron, they don't easily fit in the bins in public toilets or look that nice on. They do, however, save your life for things like camping, when no amount of prosecco or fairy lights can make you feel glampy in a wet patch. They are also excellent for hay fever and chest infections. It is soul-destroying to buy them, but they are more comfortable and effective than you'd think. Also, like Delia Smith recipes, they might *look* a bit old-fashioned, but they actually work.

But the pads and clothes (and a mini bottle of Febreze if you can find one), these are just gravy. Above *all* things, incontinence requires pragmatism, even when it feels like it will kill you. Especially when it comes to trying to sort out your body.

October 2007–July 2008, dilapidated outbuilding in the car park of a large teaching hospital, first run at fanny physio

When I return to the Australian physiotherapist who first gave me my minus score I finally find out her name – Jenny. She's pretty thrilled with the extensively detailed bladder diary I present at our second meeting and rewards me by asking me to take a look at a chart of different sizes and shapes of poo to see how mine correspond. Being constipated or having other issues may impact my bladder function, apparently. I stare at the sheet of laminated paper, headed 'The Bristol Stool Chart' (aka Bristol Stool Form Scale), in my hands. It's a neat table with illustrations of poo labelled with earthy descriptions citing texture, consistency and shape. The word sausage appears too often for me, and I feel repelled when I read 'mushy' and 'nuts'. I fumble an answer about mine being closest to a finger of fudge, reassure her I have no bottom concerns, and hope I never have to see it again.

We don't have the benefit of apps that nag you to do your exercises yet, so we have to work to a military-style timetable with encouragement/telling off from Jenny when we meet, depending on my adherence to the regime. She's my Teletubby commando,

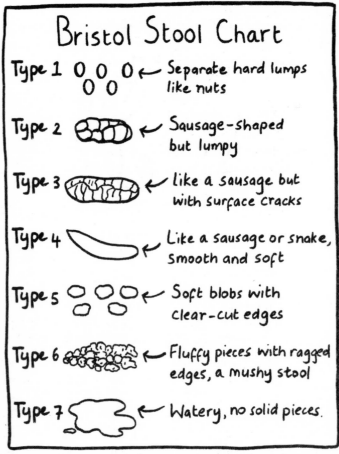

Bristol Stool Chart

Type 1 — Separate hard lumps like nuts

Type 2 — Sausage-shaped but lumpy

Type 3 — Like a sausage but with surface cracks

Type 4 — Like a sausage or snake, smooth and soft

Type 5 — Soft blobs with clear-cut edges

Type 6 — Fluffy pieces with ragged edges, a mushy stool

Type 7 — Watery, no solid pieces.

Based on Rome Foundation's original BSFS. Copyright 2000.

shouting 'again, again' as I squeeze and gurn while she checks for improvements in my strength.

As the weeks tumble into months she even makes me use fanny weights, white globules of ergonomic plastic like something Apple might sell to match your iPhone. She writes down the make of pelvic floor exercise cones on the small cardboard folded slip where they fill in my appointment dates by pen, like an old school

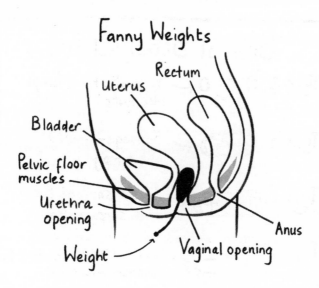

Fanny Weights

- Uterus
- Rectum
- Bladder
- Pelvic floor muscles
- Urethra opening
- Anus
- Weight
- Vaginal opening

library card. My mum has to do the ordering for me of course, as I falter at the (this time online) checkout. Again.

It turns out they are made by a French company, which gives me a boost – everyone seems to be very confident that the French know how to do it when it comes to pelvic floor exercises, providing classes after birth for all women and checking improved control as part of the sign-off criteria post-birth. I do wonder if I would have had nearly so much trouble if I'd given birth over there but eventually conclude the real benefit would be for all women to be sent the message that putting up with leaks is neither required, nor the norm.

The weights may still save me though. They consist of four silver washer-sized cylinders ranging from 5 to 20 grams, and two pellets or 'cones' which are like plastic robotic tampons or the plastic capsule inside a Kinder Surprise, but with a handy removal cord. I hold them in my palm like a jumping bean. Will they help? The case they come in is about as subtle as the ones for diaphragms and is the sort of aqua green designed to be soothing, and just off the spectrum of colours of piss. The cones come in two sizes: a large one (easier to grip) for beginners and a thinner one which is all together more tricksy and needs more strength.

It takes trial and error to find out how many grams I can lift – and resilience. If you thought minus three was bad, imagine not having the core strength to hold up 10 g for 20 minutes! As you improve, you have to experiment, making light movements and walking around without firing the bullet-shaped cone back into your knickers. But I was too squeamish for that, so I wore mine in the shower. I've also learned since that it is best to get advice before using weights of any kind at home if you might have a prolapse.

To sort my urge incontinence, which has an emotional element along with the physiological, I have to retrain my bladder, going right back to first principles, how and when and how much I pee, and what feelings I experience as I do. Jenny instigates a strict enforcement regime to quench the problem. She decrees that I can no longer run or make a special effort to get to the loo on time.

'What's the worst thing that could happen?' she asks as my face crumples at her plan for me to roll this out in the New Year.

'I piss myself in a meeting? The whole world sees my shame? I die of a panic attack in the street?' I think.

But I realise that isn't how it works.

For me, and it turns out millions of incontinent people, the triggers for *urge* incontinence are things like opening the front door, reaching the bathroom, or seeing the toilet. The incontinent leak happens tantalisingly close. You're nearly there when it all gushes out. It's also known as 'latch-key' or 'key in lock syndrome'.

You can see sufferers, usually women, scouring each new location for toilets as they arrive anywhere. It is the sort of thing that families joke about, Grandma always needing to know where the nearest loo is, people going 'just in case', but urge incontinence is a nightmare. The worst kind of nightmare as there is nothing unfounded about the fear.

You are far more prone to complete voiding (emptying) when things go south with urge incontinence than you are with simple stress incontinence (where the physical stress makes your bladder's stopper-system briefly fail). Sometimes even just the sound of turning a key can set you off – the second click in the lock is a killer. You are never, ever, home and dry.

Urge incontinence brings home the silence more strongly than anything else perhaps because psychological and physical symptoms and sensations are so entwined. Your panic and anxiety *does* set the weeing off – but you have to move beyond seeing the whole shebang as a personal failure. Also, the treatment involves not running, or giving into fear, and consequently can be a messy business at first.

But it would have felt easier, better even, if I'd met someone else who'd been through it. If I'd met someone who could say 'the treatment's hardcore but it worked for me'. If I'd had someone to swap thoughts with on laying out multiple outfits at the start of each day, or getting adult piss out of a carpet.

The retraining is a brilliant mixture of humiliation and hope. I soldier on and improve. The Kegels tone my floor, I learn to live in the no-woman's land of 'just continent enough' with only occasional accidents. I also learn a lot about urinary tract infections, which antibiotics give you thrush and what time of day the GP needs a sample by when I feel the burn. I try to be grown-up but there is a gnawing sense of something, probably disgust, or despair, that in trying to fix my continence I have wound up in a land of leaked-on pants and clothes. I am permanently on the edge of being unhygienic.

My son spurs me on. It hatches new emotions in me as he rolls and laughs and sits and stands, dribbling the forward, upward motion of his life gleefully into my mouth. And with a pang, at every milestone, his in life, mine in physio, my heart whispers temptations of a 'normal' future, where I can make plans and move on. Have another baby even.

Jenny is happy. She signs me off. I no longer have a hospital number. I'm a person again.

'Kiddo,' I think, 'we're good to go.'

July 2008–January 2009, Victorian terrace, strewn with toy buses and building blocks (for a new life)

My husband, cautious and exhausted himself, starts to share my hopes. We begin to look outwards. Maybe we can become a standard, average family. Maybe we can have a baby without time stalling at his or her delivery.

In a leap of faith he even throws away the notepad he kept in his bedside drawer all this time, the list of contraction times and scribbled notes from labour ward.

Encouraged by that act, I learn to help him, to look at him clearly and see what he has done, holding things together this whole time when I couldn't. In the early morning light we remember why we did it all in the first place. Hope, even, for the babies that we could create (spring babies, summer babies, Christmas babies). Dare to smile about the future.

Along with working like a demon on my pelvic floor, I had one other good idea that year. I decided to start talking about it a bit. I'd read enough to realise that if the statistics were true, incontinent and postnatally mad women must be everywhere. I wanted to test it out.

It wasn't easy at first and I was conflicted. I wrote to a friend:

No one talks about it and when it happens to you, well, you contrarily want to both scream it loudly in the street and never, ever, ever mention it again.

But a brittle voice told my story again and again – to my GP, to select friends, to other women in hospital waiting rooms. I no doubt scared some as I tried to work out how to connect, but I needed to make a link. I even wrote a piece for the magazine for new mums printed by a local branch of the NCT – though I didn't dare to write it under my full name. I took aim at continence myths and other sticks used to beat new mothers, especially the emphasis on gratitude – the idea that we should all be indebted to the universe even when it has served us a knackered birth canal along with a kilo of lemons. I wasn't all downbeat though; I always added a happy ending when I wrote my story, made mine an upbeat narrative arc where I got better over time.

I felt like the poster girl for post-birth incontinence in my area. Friends of friends kept buttonholing me at parties to talk about their sneezing disasters. My story was out.

Later, I discovered that the snapshot I'd thumped out over email was published in other places too, when someone I knew from university told me she'd guessed it was me from the excessive swearing, and the grisly birth injuries she'd heard about on the grapevine.

Two sorts of fame to contemplate there then, I thought ruefully. My dirty mouth remains infamous, and I *am* one of those women whose birth disaster is shared in hushed tones after all.

Chapter 9

Booze

S hallow though this no doubt makes me sound, the relationship between booze and my health woes, the fact that alcohol
made even worse my trauma two-for-one – loose bladder neck,
looser brain – was in some ways one of the hardest parts. I love
booze and booze stories. I learned to down a pint at 16 and never
looked back, so it was hard to work out what to do when warned
off it.

Unfortunately, alcohol and incontinence are inextricably
linked – anyone brought up around boozing knows getting
loaded makes people desperate for a pee and more likely to leak it
out. Ditto alcohol and depression, it's just that it is your maddest,
saddest, angriest thoughts that escape in public in a shameful way,
rather than your piss.

Harder though was seeing what happened when I ignored
those warnings. And then looking back and realising just how
much I was using booze as a way to hide my problems in plain
sight, making it difficult for people around me to see their full
impact, or do anything to help me help myself.

But just like understanding my body, my relationship with
booze started way before I ever held a real baby. Before life
presented a reckoning. Before I'd ever had a drunken epiphany.
It began when I was still on the pill, drinking cider and black, and
pretty sure all the major feminist battles had been won.

October 1995, first term at King's College, Cambridge University

I've discovered the joy of Archers and lemonade and the allure of the Ladies, where secrets slip out after dark and strangers share mascara and saliva. The best night of my life so far was on A-Level results day, necking with my boyfriend to 'Friday I'm In Love' and then hanging around in the toilets of our small town's only nightclub, smoking B&H, discussing movies endlessly and feeling like I belonged.

Toilets aren't scary. They get me in to Cambridge University as I accidentally lock myself into one the night before my interview. I wangle my way into this intellectual powerhouse by, in part, relaying the anecdote to an austere director of studies, who is trying to ask me about Henry James. I'm not drunk but I channel my drinker's raconteur spirit and make it a story. He doesn't know what to make of me and my crude description of the lav but it makes me memorable enough to get in.

Armed only with my Doc Martens, left-wing principles and a near-full collection of Wordsworth classics, I throw myself at college life. I'm enchanted and intimidated by all of it, even the loos, which are in a lavish listed building. In week two I disgrace myself by passing out in the urinal of the men's toilet at the only all-male drinking club I'm ever invited to as a 'Lady Guest'. I cry about my floppy-haired boyfriend back at home as I sit on the rough tiled floor and have to accept a kind man's offer to hook my hair out of my mouth and steer me home. Still, as we wend our way back to my digs I see another fresher sparked out with a wet patch on his trousers, being half carried, half dragged home himself. At least I didn't do *that*, I think, relieved.

I don't remember much else about my first year apart from more drunken mishaps and the shock of being stupid studying literature, a subject I was good at in school but struggle with here because I don't have a classical background (or the temperament to make up for that by studying harder in the holidays).

I spend all term panicking about getting my two essays a week in on time, and all holiday staring at the stack of *books I should have read* that is growing steadily next to my bed. I panic in listed buildings, where the paintings on the walls cost more than my mum's Vauxhall Nova. I love the books I'm reading but have no idea whether they will teach me *anything* about life. I think this is especially true of medieval poetry.

1996, Michaelmas Term as we have to call it (I know!)

Today's tutorial is with a medievalist called Doctor Nicolette Zeeman. She's a working mother with short hair and big glasses, and I like her immediately.

This week, exceptionally, I have done all the background reading, including a long raggedy pastiche by an English poet called John Skelton. It is called *The Tunnyng of Elynour Rummyng*. Until last week, I had never heard of John Skelton. This week I have a strong opinion.

The entire first section is gleefully grotesque. Elynour is 'Comely crynklyd' and 'Woundersly wrynkled', she's got a face like a pig's ear 'brystled' with hair. Her nose is hooked, her skin is slack, she is pitifully gummed, fingered and thumbed. I am unsettled by the poet's repetitive, unswerving focus on physical detail.

I think, 'I am a woman; I get drunk, perhaps in front of men who review my nose and belly and face and hair and weight.'

Elynour (or Elinor, depending on what kind of Middle English purist you are, or which copy you hastily found in the library) runs a tavern, where she sells beer full of bird shit and observes the locals. John Skelton is the sort of arse who would be writing for a gossip rag these days, I think. And he's a snob.

Apparently, the unsavoury subject affected his reputation for a while. And I concede it is probably quite brave to use the format of a prayer or liturgy but with base and informal subject matter back in Tudor times. Normally, I'd feel a kinship with Skelton for sticking it to the higher-ups and capturing the unmentionable poor. So much of Cambridge is still so aristocratic that I feel like a working-class warrior because I went to state school and my parents are under 40, even though I am palpably middle-class, privileged and not the first person in my family to go to university. But I'm too incensed with the focus on the bodily to feel solidarity with John, a laureate and advisor to King Henry VIII. I see it every week, studying English. Women presented as chattel, objects for men to criticise, conquer and own. It's the height of 'girl power' and I've read *The Female Eunuch* now. I am both raging and already bored of women being discussed in a mercantile and tawdry way. *Haven't we already protested all this shit?* I think, safe in the knowledge that female empowerment is here now. It's the '90s after all.

We isolate the worst passage. It is about a notorious woman called Alice, who rocks up and has the temerity to get drunk and rowdy. Her night out ends thus:

And as she was drynkynge,

She fyll in a wynkynge

Wyth a barlyhood,

She pyst where she stood:

Then began she to wepe,

And forthwith fell on slepe. 372-377

So, something like – 'and as she was drinking, she started winking (or closing her eyes). In a barley-hood – she pissed where she stood, began to weep, and then fell asleep'. Standard.

It's a good summary of the trajectory of feminine drunkenness, I admit. I'm a terrible winker and weeper when wazzed (though the winking reference could simply mean she's drifting towards passing out). And I love the phrase 'barley-hood', which means the sudden onset of being drunk – often accompanied by being bad-tempered. It's a neat sixteenth-century way of describing the tipping point, that mystical sip of wine too far that takes you from merry straight to battered with no in between.

Kindly, Dr Zeeman points out the sociological and historical cultural context of the poet and his work. And tells us it is supposed to be funny and show the earthy detail. I am unconvinced. At least Chaucer's famous salty woman, The Wife of Bath, has some 'oomph' to her prologue drenched in piss as I remember it. When her husband bores on at her with endless stories of shrewish and terrible wives, including Socrates' wife Xanthippe, who threw a pot of pee all over him, the Wife wreaks her own revenge and proves her philosophy that marriage works better when women rule the roost. It won't get me top marks, but I'm pretty sure Skelton is a condescending, over-literary dick-head and his poem is not very nice.

I forget about this poem for a long time, including, sadly, during my finals.

I do retain several habits learned at university for the rest of my life though – spotting my flaws but not knowing how to sort them out, leaving my clothes like a temple to the previous day's me in a pile at the end of each evening, vomming when really drunk and keeping towers of books that I haven't read yet in my bedroom.

The book and clothes piles are useful; every single day starts with a healthy dose of guilt at all the things I should have done in life, epitomised by the fact that I trip over yesterday's knickers and stub my toe on an unread copy of *Anna Karenina*.

The drinking is more complicated.

Minutes into our second meeting, while talking 'lifestyle', my post-birth physio Jenny has advised limited alcohol consumption, possibly forever, due to my broken pelvic floor. 'For ACTUAL FUCK'S sake,' I think, as soon as I hear this.

Secretly I know she's probably right, but it feels like life is heaping on the punishments and I really can't bear the thought. It stands to reason. Coffee, tea, fizzy drinks, citrus, spicy foods, and tomatoes can all make things worse, triggering new symptoms and exacerbating old ones. There's loads of science as to why. But alcohol is probably the worst (not least because of the risk of puking).

Everyone knows alcohol is a diuretic, for example, even if they can't spell diuretic and don't know what it means. In laywoman's terms, it makes you make more pee. This is not ideal when your bladder is already overstretched and overworked – the poor thing basically gets an extra load of wee to carry around. Poor boozy bladder, wanging around inside me, toppling over like an over-stretched drunk balloon.

Alcohol is a depressant too, as anyone who's shared gin with me will know. Emotions aside, even moderate usage can relax your bladder muscles, stopping them giving a fuck about the day job. As they get floppy and less into it, they open up the already fragile gateway to more leakage, and *voilà*! Mess.

Booze can also bollocks up your brain signals so you don't register quickly enough (or have the speediness of mind or body) to get to a toilet fast. This doesn't just happen to leaky people, you only have to look at all the people weeing up alleys and against trees seconds away from their house to know drunkenness enhances desperation.

Even worse, not only relaxed, receiving garbled messages and full to bloody bursting, your bladder will also be irritated by alcohol. Furious, probably. Not only is regular drinking especially problematic for people whose continence woes are related to an overactive bladder, but it makes you dehydrated, which also gets your bladder ticklish.

These facts, though obviously true, ignore the upsides. For me, over my full decade of leakiness, alcohol's redeeming features were making me think everything was screamingly hilarious, allowing me to cry and rant, thereby exorcising some grief and rage, as well as removing my inhibitions. Which meant I frequently laughed until I pissed, talked frankly about my fancy, and forgot to care about it. Until the morning at least.

And in my experience, outside building your pelvic floor to iron strength, there's little you can do about the force of pee that comes out when you vomit, apart from putting a towel between your legs and trying not to do it that often.

Sadly, for me, especially when I started drinking again post-birth, I still thought most of these were theoretical risks.

Winter 2007, *Pizza Express, a rainy evening*

Tonight is a milestone. It's my first evening out since he arrived. I am shell-shocked about my flange issues, but jam-packed with antidepressants and determination.

I have a lot of elastic, white, doughy belly to pile into my control underwear but it makes me only passably fat, and I can just about get a large Tena Lady in there. It's only one evening, and I'm not running anywhere, I think. This should be fine. And my tits look amazing. Hot cubes, bulging to busting even though I've just unlatched him, they are resplendent in an inappropriate top with a sheer layer over a fitted bodice chosen precisely because it isn't suitable for breastfeeding. 'Take that, world,' I think as I sit down for dinner. I *will* try to pretend I am the same woman I was before.

My husband, his father and his brother are all looking after the infant together. It's cute. I'm hoping my baby son won't cry all night and that if he does they won't tell me. And I feel pressure to enjoy myself. Really though, behind my brave face and fancy clothes, my arms feel empty and I miss my boy. I want to stick my face on his round belly and let him sprawl on me in a spider monkey half-hug.

I'd wonder if I will always be too stressed to actually enjoy being out, but I have another more pressing concern. It's halfway through the meal and I think my bladder neck is getting slack.

I'm trying to hide it. I'm out with old friends having pizza. Everyone is drunk and alive in the real world. It glitters. It's so loud, so fast, and so different from the new-mum world I now live in. Nobody is about to cry or fall asleep.

I wink and gurn and make an excellent series of jokes about pregnancy, labour, motherhood to an audience of women who have not yet experienced these things. I am a natural wise old hag and make them squeal about a doctor asking my husband if he'd like to look at my nicely positioned cervix. Cervix chat can get women hooting with laughter, and I can do an excellent impression of the guttural, pre-transition moo sound that signals the baby is almost here, along with the anal burp. Though I think that last detail puts them off their dough balls.

I don't mention my recent post-natal depression diagnosis as it makes me feel weird. I've only really talked about it online, where I'm anonymous, and to my middle sister, who is travelling in Australia. She rings at funny times, and often catches me tearful and off guard, in the house when nobody else is around. Speaking to her so many miles away feels a safe place to admit the truth behind all the great Facebook I am giving. I miss her, and all my sisters. I don't want to sully them given they are so young, but I want to be touched by hands that are just like mine.

I don't mention my incontinence issues either. Partly because I'm hoping I can cure it before anyone finds out. I've been doing my exercises religiously, whenever I remember I'm alive. Which is ironic because when the prosecco comes home to roost and I wet myself in the restaurant I learn incontinence really does make you feel kind of dead inside. I learn *that* at the same moment I find out what happens when one Tena Lady isn't enough.

Pop quiz. What do you think happens? A short warm burst of liquid, a drip, a squelch sound? Nope. Better. A combination of ALL THREE. And then the pad does a kind of 'roll' in my pants, it's a kayaker in peril, twisting like those fortune-telling fish from Christmas crackers. It turns over, like a stinky Quaver, like it is alive. I pray the other dinner guests will just imagine early motherhood has given me a new slightly startled resting face, and hobble to the loo, hoping the pad dumpling will not slide down my leg and end up a filthy marshmallow on the floor.

When I eventually get home my son is as beautiful as I remember, and snarls and screams and gums his way onto my bangers the second I sit on the sofa. Sweet. He's so ferocious I panic and rip my top.

Ah well, I think, realising I will have to find a way of getting my in-laws out of the lounge so I can sort out the damp patch I'm probably making on the sofa, *I probably wouldn't have worn it again anyway.*

It is only as he latches I remember I was supposed to 'pump and dump' my boozy milk. He's not impressed when I remove him and soon we're both crying. It isn't the last time I think I am the worst mother.

Spring 2009, mid-evening, a nice wine bar, centre of town

My son is older, still feeding but now walking too, and dragging me around my house, pointing out possessions I have owned for years like they are newly discovered treasures. Flicking his golden curls, he drags me forward, sharing his newfound passions: buses, lions and a film called *Cars*.

In an attempt to expand my exhausted, shrinking mind I join a new book group.

I've had all my physio and though my pelvic floor's not perfect, sometimes it is great. Other times it is not so great, like when I'm on my period, though tampons can work like pessary plugs and do you considerable favours for the first hour or two (if your insides are taut enough to keep them in place). Alcohol is still a menace, but one I've learned to live with. Needs must. I'm resigned to taking the risk of pissiness if I cane it too hard with the Sauvignon.

I'm prepared now too. Not like that ghastly first night out. Always prepared. I've got much better at knowing which brands fit me, and which clothes work over which pads without making you walk like a cowboy, so I reckon I can contain it.

I am still slightly upset about having a broken body, and crying about it a lot. But this is a new start. I am more worried about whether I'm capable of grown-up conversation; earlier today, I scolded a senior male colleague, wagging my finger in a meeting.

The new book club women don't care if I'm depressed and a bit *traumatical*, they like me anyway, and take life for what it is – frequently shit but there to be lived. They squall and laugh and shout all night. About feminism, politics, children, not having children, poetry, Jilly Cooper and vaginas. They talk about their husbands and girlfriends and partners, the good books they've read, and the bad ones. They refuse to select just one a book a month; you have to bring a pile. 'A pile!' I think. 'I can finally offload my book guilt.'

I don't break the seal until nearly 11 p.m. A triumph. Though by then I've got a new definition of 'breaking the seal'. Pre-baby it meant the dangerous act of going to the toilet during a night out drinking and thereafter needing a wee every round; now it means the first brace that doesn't work (that marks the shift to leaking with every movement and giggle that follows). On this night it happens during an impromptu round of gruesome stories starting: 'My friend, who worked in A&E …' and ending with the removal of improbable articles from an experimenter's foof. We'll come back to this later.

Once I start weeing, I decide I might as well keep drinking. I get so drunk I cry about PTSD all the way home. The taxi driver tactfully ignores even the loudest sobs.

I drop my clothes in a pile on the landing and prepare for the new staple of incontinent life, the shower before I go to bed. Standing in the steam, I realise it. Drunk as a skunk, pissed past my tipping point, having reached my 'barley-hood', I remember Elynour! And Alice! And I see that Skelton's slightly brazen women are just mums on the lash. I had the right indignant fire but for the wrong point in time, the wrong age of womanhood, so complacent was I as a young woman reading it.

I focused on Skelton's misogyny, hating on his boozehounds for their dirty skirts and their dirtier mouths. And like a narcissistic young fool I saw them as prototype Middle Ages 'ladettes' (one of the worst words of the '90s). But I missed them for what they really are. They might be *from* the Middle Ages but Alice and Elynour *are* middle-aged women for all time.

I Google it once I'm minty fresh with Original Source, which is much more pleasant now my stitches are healed, and enjoy being clean in my bathrobe, my window of happy fragrant normalness before I put my night-time 'knickers' on.

And there it is. *She pissed where she stood; Then began she to weep.*

I AM ALICE. It is uncommented on in the versions I can find online, as if it means nothing. But it doesn't mean nothing, does it? He's put it there so we can see her full humiliation. And that humiliation cows us all. Women wear odour control pants and use intimate washes and wipes they don't need because the perfume masks their shame.

'Why doesn't anyone talk about it?' I think.

I hold this troublesome thought for a long while. Years. And I keep coming back to the poem. I consider buying a volume of Skelton's poems for my urogynaecologist after my first continence surgery, but can't decide if I will seem massively pretentious.

When I start this book though I'm still wondering. I locate Nicolette Zeeman, now a Professor (Well done, Nicky!), and send her an email to ask about the poem. I apologise for bringing up a conversation we had 20 years ago as if she may remember it, and emailing her, out of the blue, about incontinence.

I am hopeful though, as she was valiantly nice to me right up to the end of my final year when I edited my dissertation by literally cutting up the drafts and sticking it back together into a better order with Sellotape, not knowing Microsoft Word 98 could do that for me.

Given that so many words for getting drunk are connected with continence (pissed, bladdered, wazzed) I'm surprised at both Skelton's frankness and all the editors 'skipping over' the drunken soaking. Surely the punning would be worth a mention? I start to think perhaps incontinence has always been in this para-doxical place – utterly accepted, completely well-known, but an ignored 'unmentionable', a dirty word we say out loud but then pretend we didn't. Has this always been so public and apparent (everyone KNOWS women, and drunks, wet themselves) but also unremarked upon, save for ridicule?

She emails me back within days, turning up references, many of which note a pervasive idea about women and water – that women have long been perceived in literature as 'leaky' vessels – softer and more permeable and expansive than men, wetter and connected to the lesser elements of Water and Earth. She adds:

> In response to your more general remarks, yes, incontinence must have been recognised and experienced then *as now*. And you are certainly right about its unmentionability … Skelton is a great place to start, precisely because he seems to observe so much (so many readers seem still to treat him merely as a misogynist 'literary' type, but the detailed observation in this text, among others, is one of its great paradoxes). [emphasis my own]

It's a sort of comforting kindness that she might have remembered my illiterate fury after all.

February 2010, a bar, any *bar*

A year later and even my poetic epiphany can't save me. Nor the lessons that came with it, about wrinkled ladies and the terrible impressions they make when bladdered.

My life is full of a strange sort of knowing disconnection and Mad Luce is in her element. I know the world, the world knows me, although the worst of me is hidden, I hope, for I am rotten and disgusting to my core. I still leak, especially if I forget to exercise. I exist, but as a phantom – fat and substantial enough to spill, fleshy and rank, out of my pre-maternity jeans but invisible enough to be scarily insubstantial. My thoughts mean nothing; my words are glassy, dangerous, volatile.

I go out for a drink, knowing it is a terrible idea. I could hate tonight, tell all, ruin lives, inflict pain. I could cast out true friendships, hang out old resentments, scream at those who've ever made me feel lucky. I could destroy so much.

My life story isn't real anymore; none of it is, despite the reality of the baby. He's there, he's real; except he's not a baby anymore. I've lost his infancy but have his early words and walking. He's the one with big boy pants now, with his belly laughs and questions from the top of a climbing frame. I'm the shit and piss and fury.

He crashes into my head, my hands, my senses, all at once. He's forcing connection, bellowing into my cheeks like Helen Keller's balloon, to make me register, acknowledge and show signs of loving him. Thank God for his persistence. When I'm with him I can, briefly, just about, be real. My days can run at normal speed. I am warm and alive. I exist! My laugh sounds normal, I remember things, and marvel at how easy it is to love him, but it is an illusion. Like Patrick Swayze in *Ghost* when he jumps into Whoopi Goldberg to kiss Demi Moore. I fear it is a trick of the light even when it feels like real life. But he's the only one, the only one who really gets inside enough to make me hot.

And when he leaves the room, is out of sight, is gone? I turn off again, and slip into automatic.

I'm so disconnected. I'm like a cipher drafted in to play me in the movie of my life. When I am not holding my son, I have no sense of taste. I look vacant because I can't hear any nuances, no music in the world for me. Colours are bleached, I have permanent pins and needles.

'Me' should be a part I was born to play (if not me, then who?) but I feel the costumes are wrong, and the trajectory and character development. Where am I going? What is the plan for me from the puppet master who's created this farce? My whole life is a backstory, isn't it? A pre-beginning, an early draft, a scatty note on the record about what happened the morning after the night before yesterday.

I sit in the pub, gulping at a large glass of white. Knowing that I'll get a headache before the bottle's finished and soon start to rub out the edges, fuzz away the sharpness of my thinking, which cuts against the dullness, and be free to let go, chattering out my angst without the need to punctuate my thoughts or make sense. I'm hoping to cry tonight, to roar it out, to let my ice-cold chest heave, imitating life, to make snot and tears to prove there's heat and mucus in my carcass. I realise this makes me sound like an attention-grabbing madwoman and yet I crave a breakdown, even public crying now. It would prove that something has happened. It would feel like a turning point; perhaps I'd be alive again if I can only weep, sob, gulp and scream a night away, howl and shout in some pub till staff are embarrassed to move us on, get walked out by someone who loves me and then comforted home in a cab.

But much as I yearn for a public punctuation, a key scene, a moment of utter despair, the 'all is lost' bit of the story arc, the 'point of no return', I do wonder if my defining moment has been and gone. Perhaps I'll never know whether I made the grade in the story of my life, maybe I've missed both my shining high point and my lowest ebb and I'm already in the final act or epilogue, the credit sequence even, the final list of names and deeds, and those I've disappointed, noted duly for the record.

I look at the friends I am drinking with. My sight is blurry. I've stopped wearing my glasses as even with them on I can't see the veins on leaves or appreciate the finer details of life. One friend smiles. She's talking about work, a funny story, something I would steal and retell in the old days – embellish, make ruder, always a raconteur. Her blonde hair hangs from her little head. With my rotoscoped view of the world, she looks to me like a dolly or an animation, but even in the dark pub, her face is real. I can see it briefly, my familiarity with it pulling her into focus. I remember the reality of it, which far exceeds any simple smudge effect I can see. It's a pretty face, with eyes the colour of puddles. It's funny, everyone notices her, but no one singles out the eyes. I file away a thought – I must tell her about her eyes. I know I was a good friend once: kind, thoughtful, listening, appreciative, attentive.

I drink more. I become the fat man in *Four Weddings and a Funeral*. I'm so very loud, so very rude, so very fat. They'll all remember me.

Crying isn't going to happen tonight. I keep drinking. I laugh and tell stories. I probably repeat myself. Funny stories. I am the social scalpel, slicing into anecdotes, personalities, famous people, books, holding up bare the rudest truths, which make sensible nice people laugh like light machine guns and feel bad later. I get drunker, though I'm still laughing, and my forehead stings and swims.

I just make my tube, or at least I am on a tube, on my way home, so I must have made it. It doesn't end happily though. In the carriage I throw up in my bag, and wet myself (of course). I'm wearing a black miniskirt and heels and I kid myself no one notices. A man comes up and offers me a mint. A mint! Maybe I am loveable after all! As he approaches, I have my wallet ready to hand over. I'm resigned to my vulnerability, and the appalling sight that I must be. I can't really care but I do apologise.

When we arrive in my station, I stand, wobbly, drooling but nearly there. I make the escalator and rise triumphant. *I will get home*. I dismount and feel a pull. I veer to the left and walk into a wall. I smash my face on a film poster and realise I am about to retch again. A guard approaches, looming. His frame is so big. He's going to arrest me or something, and I don't blame him and I don't care. Then she arrives.

She's not one of my friends, whom I've lost in the night. She is blonde, Eastern European, and young. She says to the guard, 'She's with me. We're going, yes? We're going,' and glides me to the barriers and up the stairs.

I witter a monologue, repeated sorrys, adding, 'I don't usually do this' and 'I don't know what to do'. She tells me to shut up and walks us away from the guard, the authorities, punishment, shouldering some blame for my horrible demise. She asks where I live. I hear every stranger danger warning ever given to me but I don't trust my dancing shoes and damp tights to navigate the zebra crossings, so I tell her my address.

She nods but has a condition, something we need to do first. It will make me feel better, she says. She stops to buy some Marlboro Red. I accept like a child taking a worm tablet. I know it will be too disgusting in my acid mouth but also that I cannot reject such generosity.

'See?' she says on her magnificently classy puff as I feel my chest sticking together inside. 'Much better.' I feel green.

She walks me all the way back to my front door. I'm trying not to cry on her, because she hasn't asked, and just keep repeating that I don't normally do things like this. That I have a job, a baby, a real life, I'm usually responsible, I'm trying to make plans, trying to be a person who thinks of the future.

'S'okay,' she concludes, talking over me with finality and with kindness. 'We all do this once, everybody makes a mistake, gets drunk, I know. Don't worry about it.' I toddle off and scrape my shin on my low garden wall. She redirects me to my front step. Perhaps, sensing somewhere beneath my drunk's hide and confidence that there is a real apology and sense of shame, but I guess realising that I need direction, the stranger – the kindly, youthful, angel stranger – repeats: 'Don't worry about it. 'Tis fine, Luceeeee,' then offers the killer blow: 'Just DON'T EVER DO THIS AGAIN.'

I laugh out loud like a demented werewolf. This beautiful European Millennial has offered the best life advice I've been given yet.

I text my husband to collect me from the doorstep because I can't work a key any more. He does so, dutifully, and I peel away my clothes. I rinse my mouth and hair, I wash my faggy hands. I climb into bed and wait. I'm too self-loathing to shower and give myself the cleanliness thrill. Let me shiver in my own piss, I think.

The child wakes up with a nightmare. I briefly lose my self-pity, wash my face with tears and rinse my smoky body as best I can with baby wipes. I get to him late and he has angry lips, but I become human with his touch and soothe him. He's sad and scared, but I realise what he wants. He has forgotten it is night time and wants to use his potty. Clever lad, I think, and help him be a big brave boy on the landing. His piss is a victory for us all. He's sleeping before I've carried him back to his warm dry duvet.

I stare at the ceiling and find no solace in the cracks, there's no light getting in. I hear the world wake and then I get up. Coffee burns my lips and I wince as I wash my hair. But here's the clincher: I carry on. I'm FINE.

I put on a smart dress and do my teeth, twice. Feed my son porridge, take him to nursery, kissing his face and playing peep-bo through the window.

I slide my lipstick on using my phone as a mirror and glide through the tube, the corporate day-to-day ghost of myself, a confident smile, eyeliner on, my bag and laptop ready to go. I'm almost swaggering. I brazen it out at the station and don't look at the guards, though I resolve to be extra generous whenever they are collecting for charity.

I feel shoddy but really not so bad. This is the pattern of my broken heart and broken head. I hit despair, in a bar, on the sofa, as I sit on the toilet, cry, endanger myself, spend all night worrying and then pick myself up. I attend meetings, have ideas, write reports, plan trips. I keep buggering on, waiting for something to change. I feel this strange existence may be all I get. And the glimpses of joy with my round-faced shadow, who screams with delight when I roll my terrible eyes like a Wild Thing, who keeps me human, are enough. I can live like this for him, with him, and power through the other bits, I decide.

Three days later, I find out I am pregnant.

It was only then that I started to have the uneasy realisation that this whole time, the early years, the first physio, the depression, delaying further treatment, had really just been my prep, my training. I'd polished my armour and learned my moves with the Jedi masters. But the franchise would need to be re-booted before we could see the scope of the real battle yet to come.

'Oh GOD,' I think, out loud, looking at the word 'pregnant', with all its joy and foreboding muddled together, beaming at me from the digital stick. I touch my tummy and mouth to myself, 'Everything's going to be okay, isn't it?'

I think of the first time I knew what having another baby might mean, on a bus early in my maternity leave, sober but shaken by a night of wailing colic, when an old friend whispered: 'Guess what?', her face high-pitched and all over the place. I scramble to make sure I show her I am as excited for her as I truly feel, but I'm thrown into a bundle of trauma and self-reflection.

It happens all the other times too, friends, colleagues, anyone who gives me that unmistakable smile, that flash in the eyes, a peep at a scan photo, that look which is filled with the thrumming sensation of life. I feel the hum of cells dividing and anticipation within them, I'm like a witch; but it sets off a background noise, like a caffeine-high somewhere behind my right eye. I have to check that my face is fixed right, and doesn't falter as the fear kicks in. Selfish fear, for me, I know. Selfish dread that even on hearing great news from others I am overwhelmed by my own contradictions.

I am at that stage of life, I feel like I hear this 'I'm pregnant' news every week, and I must find a way to handle it, the weird internal monologue. Hopefully most times I manage myself. Convince myself and them, if they notice, that I am pleased. That I am not growing mean and bitter, pessimistic even. It's just the two truths are there at the same time and I can't always separate them. Trauma is taunting me, echoing around my forehead. I am genuinely thrilled for all of them. The conversations and hugs, the squeals of delight, the kisses and dancing and joy and plans. I mean *them*, I feel them. It's just there is a parallel *me*, a faraway me, steeped in sensation, slinking back into the coldest corners, palms sweating, chest freezing over.

Because even in the madness, somewhere inside, my little girl dreams are still humming too. I know I want another baby, all the babies I ever did want. But will I be able to make it through the next minute, let alone 40 weeks of pregnancy again, knowing what the sound of your brain snapping sounds like, knowing what can come, and what can go wrong?

Chapter 10

Starting again

A new pregnancy means a new set of choices. Should I ask for a Caesarean section – will that be a panacea for me? There's a lot of discussion of C-sections when I talk, even in part, about my first birth story, from medical types and also other women trying to be helpful. I want advice but I don't know what to do with it and I am quite quickly confused.

The gist when I meet a new medical team seems to be that there is no reason why I couldn't have a successful, less traumatic vaginal delivery this time, especially given my tear was not extreme. The tear's impact on my life was *not* trivial, but medically, the damage wasn't catastrophic. It wasn't third or fourth degree – and it didn't take out the muscle that controls my bottom or go into the lining of my anus or rectum. I don't feel pressure to have a 'natural' birth, like that's a be-all or end-all, but everyone feels quite confident we can avoid a more medicalised delivery this time, all things being equal, which is what I desperately want. They also note that a Caesarean might damage another set of muscles and is a major operation. I realise I am terrified of being in an operating theatre too. More impersonal hands on my body. Somehow that feels worse than a lonely labour ward, the thought of such a medical place (and more people I don't know wearing masks and touching me) makes my head dance with visions of blood clots and men in scrubs rushing around. Panic is never far away. Flashbacks skitter into view, in the corner of my eye, like mice running past a skirting board. Anticipation is the enemy: the fear looms large, whenever I try to look forwards with hope. I'm pretty agitated when I arrive for my 'booking in' appointment.

Like many hospital corridors nowadays, these ones are steeped in pictures and displays showcasing the institution and its history – famous previous doctors, founders, celebrated midwives, scientists, pioneers and, occasionally, patients. As I slip in the first time, I see women everywhere looking down from the walls and get a strong sense this is the place for me, a place for a woman who will try her best not to fuck around or wallow in previous disappointment.

It's hard, though, not to be a bit weighed down by history's hands on my shoulders and I have my first full panic attack in the waiting room when I can't explain what was difficult about my first birth properly and then a midwife has to explain to me that my previous experience, and current health, mean I am 'high risk'. For me 'high risk' means no birth centre and things will likely be fairly medicalised, which is predictable but hard to swallow.

I weep on the chairs in the busy waiting room and am somehow scooped up by a senior midwife, who guides me into an office and gives me three things. A pat on the shoulder, a glass of water and the on-the-spot promise that she'll be part of my care team. A face to recognise. An anchor. I think perhaps she senses the shock in my face, can see my terror, though maybe she just wants to move me somewhere quiet so the other patients aren't traumatised by my ragged breathing.

This fear sets the tone. The trouble with a traumatic backstory is that I can't leave it behind. My second pregnancy can't be as positive as I want it to be. It can't be a form of 'moving on', because it's endlessly defined by discussing that first birth with new people. By May, I've talked through my first son's birth five times: to a psychiatrist, a psychologist, a frosty but helpful consultant and two midwives.

The second midwife I tell cries when she hears my story in full. I thought it would be too common-or-garden and then realise suddenly as I'm telling it, that that's the point. The mundanity did her in in the end, mine is just another story of disempowerment. Casual indifference to the person giving birth, which even kindness at the end couldn't undo, and which caused lasting injury and unnecessary damage.

She dries her eyes and works to erase some of the self-blame I carry around like hot sand in my chest, to challenge my conviction that if I'd only handled my first labour better, I could have avoided my complications. She focuses on helping me process my bad birth, rather than offering a magic bullshit-bullet by guaranteeing a better second one. It seems like tough love, but she's scathing about all the people who've suggested circumstances or my actions within them could have changed my fate, however much they were trying to help. She says nobody, least of all midwives or healthcare professionals, should be saying that things like a water birth may have prevented my specific damage and its ramifications.

'It seems to me you are blaming yourself for the fact that you had a tear,' she adds, in an email about what choices are available for me when it comes to my second delivery. She stresses it was not my fault and repeats that it is extremely common to have some degree of 'perineal trauma' in a first delivery. It's striking, hearing it so baldly stated, with such clarity, from someone who has only met me a few times, but she's right.

It's not the most empowering thought ever, but it helps in a funny sort of way. Maybe I couldn't have done it all so much better after all.

Late July 2010, large shiny hospital, looking overdue though I'm not even halfway through yet

My body, the cheeky bastard, has decided to imply to the world that it is good at pregnancy and babies. Before I even wash my hands from my pregnancy test it flexes out into a bump. I can't keep it quiet while I get used to it. I know the bump is probably wind but to others it's *evidence* of the new thing.

Whatever causes my immediately fertile figure, it has the force of military spec anti-bladder training. My muscles give up the ghost the second they have a foetus to blame for their laziness.

My midwife sends me to physio. I do not realise this will become my second home and head down to the offices with interest, clutching onto the thought that I couldn't have prevented my injuries.

My instinct to apologise for flooding is strong. I try to practise saying 'It is not my fault' but I'm not convinced.

The therapist is also pregnant with her second baby. I recognise the world-weary look, tired pale face, and the noise all the fibres in her body are making. Like mine, her body tingles with a sarcastic shrill of 'AGAIN? WHAT A *FUCKING IDIOT.*'

Given my history it is no surprise that things are collapsing, she says, but she can't examine me due to infection risks.

I'm disappointed. I am scared I'm not doing enough because I can't really feel the exercises properly anymore and everything, including my pelvis, feels loose.

'I can't feel the pull even when I really gurn,' I say. 'Can you check if I'm doing them right?'

She tells me to check myself. But I'm nonplussed. 'I haven't been trained,' I say. 'I don't know what to look for.'

'You have fingers, don't you?' she points out. 'You can feel it.'

I think, 'Won't that be a little bit like … *wanking*?' But decide to see how it goes; maybe if I use my own hands to check if I'm on the right track I can plough on, sensation be damned, and then come back after I've given birth.

I clench in the lifts out of the basement, though not with a hand in my pants because PUBLIC, and assume I won't be back there until after the baby is born. We all know what assume does, to you and me.

That summer I lose my optimism. Panic sets in and I am diagnosed with PND's shameful little sister Antenatal Depression (AND). I know I should be happy, but I am retreating from my life again. Crying. Not sleeping. My husband's starting to look pretty tired, and he has a transport-obsessed three-year-old to worry about too.

I hide in the bathroom at night, convinced I'm going to die. I can't think or talk about death out loud, not when the toddler might be listening. But can I survive at all if death is all I can think about?

I realise that we can't do this on our own, not this time.

September 2010, lounge floor strewn with toy vehicles, a small boy watching bus rallies on YouTube

Our doula, Mars, a woman whose job it is to help women, and their partners, through birth, rocks up at our house in a royal blue dress with her eyes full of starlight and good sense, and the air of Mary Poppins, if Mary Poppins spoke more lovingly about amniotic fluid, vaginas and the healing power of red wine.

She wants to know our whole family if she is to be a part of it and help us. She meets my toddler first, who explains carefully to her that I am having a baby, another boy, but then makes it clear he'd rather talk transport. She makes an impassioned plea for the number 9 bus as superior to the W3 with our son, and then listens to my husband and me recount his birth. It tumbles out in a paranoid jumble. My trauma snapshots and my husband's. Things I'd forgotten. After-effect after after-effect.

She stays calm when we get shaky and lets us get it all out. When we finally finish she smiles and says: 'It would be an honour to be at his brother's birth.'

From the minute she says that, I feel better. Only a tiny bit better – I'm still poorly mad – but better all the same. And sometimes just a tiny bit of better has to do. Like when a few weeks later I reach crunch point and my pelvis collapses. And I find to my cost that your pelvic floor muscles do more than keep your pee in place – they hold your whole body and life together.

Chapter 11

Pelvis

'You never think it'll happen to you' is a well-worn defensive cliché. We all know it, we all think it won't happen anyway. And I'm not necessarily against it. In its own way ignoring reality can help against the temptation, in the face of all the evidence that shows life is a colossal arse, to curl up in the foetal position and refuse to engage with anything.

But with Symphysis Pubis Dysfunction (SPD – now referred to as Pelvic Girdle Pain (PGP)) – I did something worse than bury my head deep down in the desert. I knew it *could* happen to me. I'd had symptoms in my first pregnancy, some nagging pain, mostly relieved by paracetamol and rest, and been told I would have a predisposition if I ever got pregnant again. I just somehow thought I didn't *deserve* it.

PGP is the umbrella term for uncomfortable and painful symptoms around your pelvis. SPD is one condition covered by that umbrella. Health professionals tended to describe it to me as a separation at the front of my pelvis due to pregnancy hormones loosening all my ligaments, including those which kept my pelvis together. The pain is caused when the symphysis pubis – the place where the bones at the front of your pelvis meet – widens and/or becomes unstable and uneven. It can happen to anyone, though is most common in pregnant women.

My shock on getting it again wasn't because it was unbelievable, but because it felt like such a fucking swiz.

Pelvic Girdle Pain (PGP)

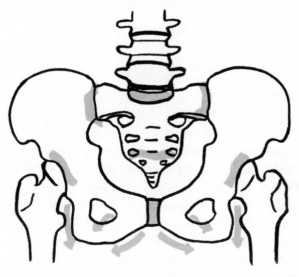

= Pain experienced around the pelvis

For me, it starts with twinges and the feeling I've been kicked in the girl space so hard I am vibrating with the force. It gets worse over several days. Suddenly, climbing motions – up stairs, onto buses, into a bath – make me hurt as well as leak. My centre of gravity begins to slide.

It is distracting but so is life. I have a list of things to do with my boy in our last season of the Mummy and Me show. Like visiting the London Transport Museum. How painful *can* climbing onto a twentieth-century tram be? I have a blinding shock as I attempt it and have to hobble home. Spreading my legs wide enough to walk smarts. Online advice includes measuring my ankles and knees at the point before it hurts the most with a length of string, then taking that length of string into labour with you and using it as a guide so no one wrenches your thighs too far apart.

Mars says she will take charge of that and I can just concentrate on keeping well.

October 2010, getting ready to go to work in an office block, with four floors

'They will probably just tie me back together with elastic,' I joke to my husband, who is leaving to fly away for business for a few days. I have an appointment coming up to sort my sore bits, and as I kiss him goodbye, I just repeat my mantra 'It's all going to be okay though, isn't it?'

I'm still hoping for the best as I head off to work.

It is the worst kind of insanity, this calming down and carrying on, as it comes from the last fragile dregs of optimism I have left.

I manage to get my son to nursery, because we have several stops to admire the bendy buses. But as I walk to the tube I notice I'm resting between bursts of walking. Like I am a very old, or a very sick, person. Commuters are unusually willing to share their seats.

I pull myself along on an escalator unsure I'll ever get off, hold the sides of the lift at my office as the upward motion sends my pain into orbit, and, finally, see sparks when I try to stand up from my swivel office chair, and I realise I can't stand or walk.

Humiliation doesn't cut it. I have to be *carried out of my fourth-floor office* by a colleague and escorted to hospital.

'Good fucking God,' I think.

The hospital staff and other patients are transfixed as I try to move into the waiting room (though maybe it's the sounds I am making). A new fresh-faced physio confirms my fears, takes one look at me, agrees I can't walk, and fetches a wheelchair. I ramble incoherent thoughts like: 'Will it be okay?', 'This is worse than labour', 'Did I log off my computer?', 'What's for dinner?' and 'Who is going to do nursery pick up?'

Now I can tell you the answers were No, Hmm, Yes, Codeine, and one of my brilliant little sisters, who drove halfway down the country to work with an army of friends to keep my life afloat. But the poor colleague sitting next to me at the time can't answer. He's only offered to help me in and out of a taxi. He gives me a reassuring nod when we are sent to the labour ward for observation, accepting, or possibly not realising, that everyone in the waiting room not only assumes he's my partner, but also thinks he is a massive bastard for not holding my hand.

My pelvis, it turns out, has separated and become totally unstable. I feel like I can make out the imbalance if I touch the bony bit between my legs, though the pain is exquisite, so I don't do it for long. I spend the evening in a labour ward, and the next month getting progressively more disabled. I need crutches and have to wee in the back garden or stay upstairs all day. We set up a bed by the landing for me to lie on. The physiotherapy teams spent hours massaging and manoeuvring me from lying to sitting to standing, reminding me how to walk again. There's nothing anyone can do when the jolts of pain make me pee. Another kick in the face for incontinent people, although it's never spoken about: different bits of your body spasm in pain and, yup, your bladder joins in.

As I stand over my makeshift bucket toilet in the first frost of November I want to hope for the best. I look to the grey bright sky.

'Seriously though,' I ask, 'what fresh hell on Earth can labour bring to top this?'

Part Three

ROUND 2 – BACK FOR MORE

Chapter 12

Childbirth – Again

It takes 30 minutes in a delivery room for my second son to arrive. Perhaps there are no words for the magic of a second coming. The old newness of an echoed face, the truth, horror and surprise of a familiar wound reopened.

November 2010, labour ward, shiny hospital, fresh from a mad taxi dash across town

I am with my husband and Mars. She holds me as we stop in the corridor every few paces with my escalating contractions. Mars has faith. In women. In the wisdom of our mothers and grandmothers. In stories and female voices, and, absurdly, in me.

'You will be magnificent,' she says, as we start to walk again. 'You will do this.'

I feel pumped. Almost.

My mum texts: 'Good luck, sausage.' I am going in.

A midwife measures me and declares I am only 1 cm dilated. Her colleague asks if I want to go to the shops. And I thought being carried out of an office was humiliating.

I stomp into the en suite shower room as my son's head is now so far down into my pelvis that it locks it back together by jamming the joints like a cork.

'I want a Caesarean,' I demand. My husband tries to point out they won't do it but I just hiss, 'I'm pretty fucking persuasive.'

He dares to suggest that maybe I'm not as far along as we'd hoped. That perhaps we panicked like our taxi driver speeding down the ring road at 70mph, scared my waters would flood his back seat, but I can't be easily calmed.

The midwives take the forms away and say they will give us a minute.

'I really don't understand,' I gasp/whine through another contraction, but somehow I don't have the stomach for a fight, or, I realise, to walk as far as the door, so I sort of collapse onto the bed and start to cry. This was my chance for a formative, healing, baptismal moment. The life-changing, mythical second birth (that anyone with a shitty previous labour or delivery (or both) can only dream of). That thought is a pointless torment for me, right to the end.

A minute's self-pity is all I get though.

I feel myself bend and announce: 'My waters just broke.'

My husband and Mars are still wondering how to get me to leave.

Nothing happens. They both stare nervously at each other, and look at my legs, then each other, and then back at me, presumably thinking, 'Oh God, she's actually mad.'

I doubt myself, a second goes by, inside me a voice questions my very being. I felt so certain …

But then we're off. Slop explodes, hot all over me and the paper sheets. I am a prophet, not a fantasist. My remaining waters slurp out, slowly. Hot syrup full of meconium, filling the space between my legs. Mars hits the alarm and sprints. I can hear her feet on the corridor. She's shouting. Calling the first midwives, grabbing a doctor walking past, insisting they take charge and listen.

The alarm drones. People keep arriving. Faces round a royal deathbed. I've been this woman before. I'm not stupid. I try to close my eyes and drift but it is too urgent and swirly this time. A sea of arms open my legs, move me around the slushy bed.

I call above the din a handful of questions and apologies: 'What's happening? I'm sorry. Can I sit up? I can't stop. I don't know what I'm doing.'

'Just keep doing it,' the midwife who seems to be in charge shouts back, which feels like a riddle. Someone in blue calls to her across my belly: 'No one has told her,' and then she locks eyes with me and says: 'You're about to meet your baby.'

Mars squeezes my hand. I feel safe. My husband touches my shoulder. I feel love. But I'm still confused; this can't be it. This is just one long, tense contraction and a sensation of panic between my thighs. I'm sprawled on the end of the bed. I'm not pushing, I'm slipping. There are hands and arms all over me, moving my limbs. I don't know which ones go with which doctor. But no one else is confused, they are serious now, polished and quick, a team. The midwife's gloved hands are out, she's calling up between my legs, pleading with me to stop and pant.

I think, 'Stop what?', but I sort of judder instead and say, 'Can somebody please help me out?'

And then I see and feel and hear him all together. Our beautiful stone-grey boy. Real. Alive. Solid. Out. Out and born. And all I can say, all I can think is, 'I don't understand what's happening,' and stare at the shiny blue cord lasso twisted all around him.

But he is hot and slippy on my chest, turning pink, in seconds, nude and perfect as the arms get their act together and help me sit up. Zero to 10 cm in less time than an episode of *EastEnders*.

The midwife is as shocked as I am. 'You were only 1 cm,' she says.

Mars looks over with precision.

'Congratulations,' the midwife adds.

It is so precipitous I am briefly a celebrity on labour ward. But there's something deeper to it. The speed was us. His need to be out, my need for it to end, our need to stop everything and start it up again in one moment. He and I: we needed birth to be what it is in its purest form, an ending *and* a beginning.

Even the terror of the cord tied round his neck and body can't keep our spirits down for long as my boy is so, so lucky to be unharmed. His corkscrew of gristle didn't stop his spinning into the world like Superman. He's everything. Identical to his brother, but himself. A game changer. A star. Uninterested in the past, bellowing into the afternoon.

And my body has learned one lesson at least: my placenta flies out, intact, in a burp of fury. It bounces. None of us wants any of that nonsense again. Mars says the placenta is beautiful and life-giving. I still decide not to look.

I need stitches though, of course I do. My perineum stood no chance in the rush. But even that has benefits. I learn more about my anatomy than ever because when I finally look away from my boy's face I'm greeted by the clear sight of my now twice haggard nether-land being sewn back into place, in a crystal-clear reflection on an unfortunately placed resuscitation cot with mirrored sides. It is bloody and strange and mesmerising, a sticky red cave of brokenness. I am briefly entranced, so many flaps and craggles, and so covered in bright, glowing red blood, before it makes me almost faint and I ask politely if they can cover up the mirrored surface.

'Oh God,' says the midwife, realising that I cannot be the first woman with a birth injury eyeful. 'You really can see everything. Sorry.'

They place a blanket over the cot and I get back to gas and air and going into shock at the strange turn of events. The midwife gets back to her extensive embroidery and says they will see what they can do to change the room set-up. Mars puts some chocolate in my mouth and strokes my forehead, letting me shake in her warm, safe hands as my husband holds the baby tight to his chest. I close my eyes and hope I don't jog the needle.

It is done.

If my second birth was an easy sequel, then the recovery was a saga. New exercises, new fanny gadgetry, but some things never change. My placenta might be out but everything else is mashed.

Chapter 13

Physiotherapy

The term physiotherapy dates back to the nineteenth century, though the process of physical touch and re-education is much older. Some health historians trace it to the Ancient Greeks, who used massage and other physical cures. Now, physiotherapists combine exercises, posture help and realignment, massage, movement, guidance, advice on how to incorporate their ideas and suggestions into your life, and endless repetitions of key exercises.

Women's health physios are often the first line of defence for continence issues. For many, physio represents a cure or huge improvement, obviating the need for more invasive surgery or procedures. It's usually quick too. My long-winded experience is not typical.

Physios who work in gynae specialisms have a particular rep for being hardcore, perhaps because they have to be brutally honest in assessing our most private parts. There is no point in them not telling you the truth, or hiding things from you, just as it will not work if you hide things from them. To help you, they need to know exactly the state you are in. It can feel like a real piss take, to have to reveal yourself completely. However, though womanning up felt like a leap of faith, it helped me and was definitely worth it.

The Swedish used to have the best name for physios: *sjuk-gymnast*, or 'someone involved in gymnastics for those who are ill'. I love this but prefer to think of them as angels. Unflappable fingersmiths unflustered by a fanny fart before their first cup of tea in the morning.

They have to be prepared to get their (gloved) hands dirty and make you feel okay about it. And bear in mind the myriad reasons why the women in front of them may well not want to be there at all.

I think they manage this because they have to listen, check progress, take notes, and bear in mind the everyday details as well as the medical minutiae. Their work cannot exist in a sterile vacuum, like hi-tech surgery. It is all about you, your body, how you use it, and how you understand it. It might also be because, when it comes to their fiddliest work – fitting pessaries, feeling prolapses, touching and watching the muscles/bulges/scars – they sometimes learn, or so they've told me, *by practising on themselves or each other.*

The physicality of physio is what most people think of, tough taskmasters encouraging people to take their first steps after an accident, use artificial limbs, get out of bed. And there is an element of force and motion, even with fanny physio, but it is on a micro level of fiddling and tweaking.

The exercises we do today are inspired by US gynaecologist Arnold Kegel, who dedicated decades to developing non-surgical methods for improving his patients' pelvic floors. He understood the trickiness of intricate movements – and solved it in 1951 by inventing the perinometer, a tool which allowed patients and doctors to see movements and objectively assess and rate muscle strength. He's the source of my bad marks right at the beginning! I never used a biofeedback instrument like Kegel's but many do, both in hospitals where physios use probes that show patients how they are doing – and with devices you can buy and use at home.

Physios working on improving pelvic floor muscles today still focus on movements inside you. And they often use metaphors first off to help you get your exercises right, telling you to imagine you are holding in a fart in front of the Queen, for example, or asking you to pretend you are trying to pick something up with your fanny.

Enacting these make-believe fanjo feats for an audience can feel like being propelled into a filthy re-hash of *Whose Line Is It Anyway?*, but these tiny squeezes, these mini-motions, are how you relearn your body. And that is a hell of a thing: to introduce someone to their new normal (temporary or permanent), and not let the moment overwhelm either of you.

The night before my second course of physio I am terrified. My eight-week-old son is in his own world of minuscule milestones and movements (holding a finger, smiling, watching the world). He's a tiny sparrow reaching out for love, but not to me; he has a higher god, his small eyes tracking his brother's every movement.

I don't want to re-enter the world of the perpetual patient. I want to lie on the floor blowing his face so he blinks and smiles, to watch my boys connect and heal the fragments.

But mostly, I don't want to know my score.

January 2011, large shiny hospital, broken-lady clinic

I shared my flange physio fears on my new blog last night. Came out as 'an incontinent'. Everyone said I was brave. I'm not brave. I have performance anxiety so strong that I am having to stare forwards and pretend I am somewhere else just to avoid grabbing my bag and making a run for it, pissing my way down another hospital corridor.

Given my close-up view of the damage, I fear I am broken beyond repair, that my fanny is finally kaput. The midwife from our home team was certainly aghast. There was no missing the incontinence this time.

I worry I'll be accused of wasting a space, bringing this on myself by having another baby at all – a familiar voice in my head snarls on repeat, 'What did you *expect* to happen, Luce?'

The negative spiral is inviting and I'm about to tumble down the rabbit hole completely when *she* arrives and stops my turmoil in its tracks.

A blonde vision called Lizzie calls my name from the end of the corridor. She's Betty Draper. She's so pretty she probably smells like freesias. I'm scared that showing her my filthy state will be some kind of blasphemy. I stare at her. Young, beautiful and neat, she is the reception teacher you would create if it was entirely up to you. She's my Miss Honey.

She knows how to keep the whole appointment on track even though my voice is shaking. She even knows when to look at me, and when to look away, when I cry.

My witty defences are out in force as I clench and cough my way through an examination, explain how pad-tastic I am, and how often I go to the loo. She seems to understand the extent of the problem from the contradictory truth: 'everything' makes me leak, and also, sometimes, 'nothing' does.

I wait for her verdict, back in my clothes, Tena-ed up and ready to go.

She scores me two.

'Get the fuck in!' I shout.

She graciously explains that minus numbers are no longer used as they were confusingly applied. My two is helped (or hindered, who knows?) by grade inflation.

'Minus numbers are so disheartening,' she adds.

Too true.

Lizzie, it turns out, is an optimist too. She's hopeful this will only take six or seven months because I have responded to exercises before.

I don't know if this is because I actually do them. Women are not always compliant with physio exercise programmes, maybe because they are a drag, or the ones with young kids barely get a moment to themselves; maybe because they are embarrassed to focus on sensations 'down there', or think they won't work; because they can't see the effects of the exercises as they do them;

or maybe because they don't think they deserve any better as life has been one long trajectory of gunk in their knickers anyway.

She also talks about my age and other women in my family, and says she'd like to refer me to a gynaecologist when things have improved a bit.

I look up. I'm not sure about that.

She reassures me they have plenty of tricks up their collective rolled-up sleeves. But she takes it slow, says it will be just to talk about the future and what could be done, or might be advised, as I grow older (inevitable), hit the menopause (likely), have more children (unlikely).

Last time the idea of planning for future problems would have seemed horribly like giving up. This time I feel that maybe if I struggle to control something so normal most of us forget we're doing it, planning is a good idea. So I leave happy. Ready to clench and report back.

But as I hit the pavement, I get the continence care kickback.

The ease with which people talk about leaking down in the clinic creates an echo chamber of empowerment. I leave thinking I am going to be immune to feeling rank. That I am going to be braver about talking about it, get 'me' back, be confident, and optimistic. And it lasts all the way up the stairs. But then I hit the street outside and the clouds start to circle. Because I know in real life, outside the comradery and destigmatising care, it will be a disaster if I fart or pee in front of everyone.

Summer 2011, a new moment of toilet shame as I get ready to go back to work for the second time

My physio is ongoing. I haven't improved in the timescales hoped for and I'm wishing I hadn't told anyone about it on my blog. I feel like I've let the side down, that I'm not trying hard enough, like I'm in Weight Watchers but eating all the pies on the sly. I'm failing at flange flexing.

In a metaphor for my stalling I am struggling to get off the toilet today. I don't have a new problem down there, but my children have crammed me into our little WC, the eldest because he wants to talk about wild animals and *Ben 10* and the youngest because he has insisted on being breastfed so strongly I've plugged him on despite being on the loo as the crying was making me nervy and my urge incontinence twitch.

I'm disconcerted to see how big the baby pawing at my knockers actually is. His growing proves our time is running out, our number's up; soon, I'm going to have to go back to work. It makes me gulp, to be going back to work, again, still incontinent, again. Leaving behind my second small baby in the name of liberation, buggering on and two-income mortgages.

It isn't the job, or the people, that bother me. It's the vulnerability. My credible fear that shame or physical inadequacy will take over. However well-prepared or put together you are, you, as an incontinent adult, are always just one false move away from losing everything. A stair taken too quickly, a coughing fit, a jolt in the lift, an overrunning meeting and I'm not Luce Brett, the professional, I'm *that* girl in assembly again.

I've packed my bag. It includes a complete change of clothes and some baby wipes, a long cardigan, pads and a hospital letter for my next appointment to show to HR. By Christ, I'm bored of my incontinence outfit by now. I chuck in a new red lipstick though. I can be positive about change.

More importantly, I've dusted the 'lines' about being a working mother. They are my new armour, along with the flange jokes, that let me say I still have a hospital number without crying in public.

I have gooey quips, like how he needs to learn there's more than one way to sing 'The Wheels On The Bus' (even though mine is best as the driver shouts 'no more pushchairs'). And nursery will be able to teach him something I can't – that he is not the centre of the universe, even if he's the centre of mine. There are the standard lines about quality time and my mother working when we were young and it being inspirational. And then the facts. The stupid bald facts, like we could not afford for me not to work, even if most of our money is hoovered up by childcare fees.

If those lines don't work when people interrogate my 'choices' or commiserate, which both risk waterworks, then I laugh it out. 'I'm looking forward to drinking a cup of tea while it's hot,' I joke. 'And some me time.'

Depending on company, I might add 'in the eight years on my current job, no one has sucked my tits while I was on the loo. Yet.'

I get far more nods of agreement from other parents for the line about a pee break than a tea break. Even from my own mum, who arches her eyebrows. Usually when I tell a crude joke in front of her she tells me off. This time she grimaces in recognition.

I wonder why that is now that I actually do have someone sucking my boob on the toilet. I have plenty of time as he's suckling but asleep and if I wipe, I'll wake him ...

Perhaps this is because the boundarylessness of pregnancy, childbirth, then having a baby is so startlingly acute and shocking that it never leaves you. My mum had four of us, including two at once, taking one side each of her body. The public ownership of women's bodies starts with the rules on what you can put in and out of your body when pregnant – from alcohol to cheese – and the endless observation about everything from bump size to whether your hormone-drunk face is glowing or there is anywhere left on your body not covered in hair. But it doesn't even end with the violation and ruin that birth sometimes wreaks on your privates. From their first breath, our children's uncompromising view that they alone own our bodies is quite something.

Young children's love is rampant physicality. When they are tiny they think you are the same thing – you and them, mother and child, one big fuzzy, squashy over-tired motherchild. They are far worse than nurses and doctors for seeing your body as an object, *their* object.

As babies and as toddlers my sons are always sticking my fingers in their mouths and theirs into mine, casually leaving a little hand in my cleavage, absentmindedly pawing my décolletage while reading or chatting or watching TV. They touch me and rub me, grab handfuls of me. They shove and lick and stroke and pull. Both have bitten me. One so badly, and on the boob, that I had to go to an NHS Walk In Centre. Unfortunately, because I was working in the centre of London the nearest one was in Soho, whereupon I was asked by a nurse if I had sustained the human bite from a client at work.

They are the same with the house. My house is their house now. My poor house, which like my tits was once a monument I decorated to show the best of myself and my taste, is now tattered and beleaguered and prematurely aged.

They roam it like their territory. Walk in on me naked in the bath, and bump into me as if my body is a permeable ghost they can charge through. They literally ignore any sense of my space like they can't see it. My bed, my arms, my head – all belong to them and I cannot go for a wee without someone squeaking or squalling or unleashing an avalanche of 'WHY's. Leading me back to the joked-about sacred peace of a cubicle at work.

'Oh GOD,' I think with a flash of shame. The last time I stayed at my parents' house I walked into my mum's bedroom and shouted through to her in her shower room as I blundered around, looking for some nail scissors. It is such a mundane, commonplace moment, a non-anecdote, that I almost miss the importance. But I am the same as my kids. In fact, I'm worse, as I am a mum and I should know better. My mum is in her fifties. All her children are adults now. But her personal space, her body, her bedroom, her moment on the loo? Bah. It barely exists in the mind of me, her child. I cross state lines with the enthusiasm of a toddler when it comes to my mother's privacy: even 33 years into parenting she still can't have a piss in peace.

No wonder she went to work.

September 2011–May 2012, Lizzie's office, again and again and again

Over months and months of appointments I stick with Lizzie, or rather she sticks with me, as other people in my life move on.

My children are in nursery and in school. This is an amazing moment. The tick-tocking of time is harsh proof that life marches on. A small earnest boy with curly locks and a brand-new jumper edges cautiously, book bag too big, into a world where he will be his own self and I can't take care of him. It's devastating but incredible and I well up as he and his pint-sized friends marvel at the sand-pit and learn new words like register. Both boys get daily progress reports, termly updates. These are amazing, but emphasise the sour truth – my school reports are rubbish, because my life is stuck.

The baby who changed my world now uses cursive letters. His brother's finger paintings cover the fridge. Yet me and Lizzie, the physio dream team, both adults, we are *not* progressing. The only gold star we'd get is for attendance.

My twat is still not *all that*.

Lizzie chivvies. If I keep improving then I'll be able to run for a bus without leaking! I can't even rage about this fucking bullshit as it is just the truth. My new normal is just mediocre progress. Endless crappy 'improvements' as I limp on miles behind the pack.

There are some jokes. I can still PMSL. My SPD pelvis is on the mend, and the advice is 'don't spread your legs too far'. I cackle caustically for what feels like 15 minutes at the thought of ever entertaining another pregnancy.

But my muscle strength is still only two and a half. Just like in my first labour I 'fail to progress'.

Lizzie says I'm being harsh.

'Luce,' she points out, 'if you weren't in trouble, you wouldn't be here.'

Rattled by the idea of being 'in trouble' I realise there's noth-ing for it but to embrace my inner Tigger and at least accept

Lizzie's suggestion that together we explore other options. I don't know if it is hope or denial but I am certain I can do it, if I try just a bit harder.

We look at pessaries and other devices in a catalogue of doom filled with plugs and bullets and other monstrosities and I actually flinch. Later, I will come round to them, but right now sticking something that looks like a baby teether up my vagina each day seems like the last thing I can consider.

Lizzie broaches other health niggles that are making things worse, like Vitamin D deficiency and fatigue. She encourages swimming and Pilates but warns me off running, which blows, as literally everyone I know seems to be training for a 10K. Unable to do quick-fix exercises, I feel absurdly isolated in the mid-thirties push for fitness and scared I will get huge and fat and people will think that's why I leak.

My heart is on sinking sands.

As monthly, bi-monthly, 12 weekly sessions drift by, I am outraged at the cost of all the pads I'm using; I have panics when I run out and need to use two of the slim ones together. I fear them smelling if it is hard to get away during meetings or they get wodged up my bum by an unexpectedly ferocious spurt.

By the winter, when my second son is one, I am flat; by the end of the next spring, I am looping round the twist. We are talking about coffee and alcohol when I slip up and accidentally tell Lizzie too much. I don't know why I do it.

I tell her about my work Christmas party where a combination of heels, free-flowing prosecco and an ill-advised group selfie sets me off so badly I find I am standing in the middle of a busy restaurant in a large puddle, my legs warm with piss. I cover by throwing my wine glass on the floor so forcefully that splinters and shards distract everyone. I create a bubbly splash-back to re-soak my legs and mask the smell. Better to be a klutz or pisshead than an incontinent, I reason, help mop it up and toddle off in my squelchy shoes. I often do that, play the clumsy lush, I add, to explain better to Lizzie, who has gone quiet.

She looks into my soul, I think, and the room lurches. We're in a poltergeist movie and the temperature has dropped. I can hear us breathe. I worry I've offended her or she will suggest AA. Or that by telling her I still go to parties I have proven I'm doing okay and don't deserve help. Or she really hates people who waste white wine. I probably got carried away and swore too much in the retelling. I've not been victim-y enough.

'Luce,' she says, 'I've been thinking for a while that we really are coming to the end of the road.'

My stomach sinks. It jolts like a broken lift. My heart races. I am *being dumped*. Oh GOD.

'No. No. I'm sorry. I really am trying, I promise,' I blurt. Tearful, pathetic, pleading. I'm desperate though. If she dumps me, where will I go? I will have failed this too and will be stuck in my own piss forever. It is lonely enough now, with an appointment only every couple of months and someone who properly understands. Without this, I will never survive.

'Luce,' she repeats, 'Luce.'

Like I'm a baby to be soothed.

She knows how hard I've worked, she says, but she thinks we need to be honest and consider other options. She will speak to the multidisciplinary team about me. I'm only 34 but the party has convinced her. She knows that this can't carry on, and neither can I. She's not rejecting me – she's offering new hope.

I think, 'Hooray, I might be fixable.'

And also, 'Shit, I don't want fanny surgery. I don't want a knife up there. It doesn't sound very nice. Will they force me to have a hysterectomy? Whisk it all out? And what's a multidisciplinary team when it's at home? HOW MANY MORE PEOPLE ARE GOING TO LOOK UP MY SKIRT? WHO ELSE WILL SEE MY SHAME?'

Chapter 14

Urogynaecology

The multidisciplinary team is a group of different specialists pooling knowledge and expertise to improve 'patient outcomes'. They are led by an earnest consultant with expertise in incontinent women and fixing them, and they *do* almost all get to look up my snatch one way or another. Lizzie has introduced my case to the team and assured me they plot all day making broken fannies (and their owners) better again. Hurrah.

Urogynaecology is a mash-up of two areas of medicine: Urology (which looks at the urogenital system including bladders, kidneys, prostate, etc.) and Gynaecology (female reproductive organs and areas). As far as I can tell these groups share a passion for helping keep the good stuff (organs and part of your body) in and letting the bad stuff (wee) come out *but only when you want it to*. Sometimes these departments are called Female Pelvic Medicine and Reconstructive Surgery, which sounds far more frightening.

As 'conservative measures' (now known as non-surgical measures) – physio, exercises, losing weight or altering diet – are no longer working for me, my team will have to ask: is this woman a suitable candidate for surgery, and if so, which one?

For me the questions are different. I want to ask: How will I cope with a trip even further along the corridors of shame? What the hell happens down there? Do the doctors and nurses think we are a bunch of moaning smelly ladies? What did they say about me in their meeting? And how will I hold my nerve if the appointment goes badly?

I don't know if I have the stamina to admit the shameful, tedious truth again. Or to confess I haven't looked up a single thing about operations, and have avoided all mentions of the mesh scandal (discussed further on pp. 152–157), a medical saga that has been rumbling on for a while now, because I am paralysed with fear about being chopped up. And what if they can't even help me despite their expertise? What if they send me home with a shrug and I'm stuck like this forever?

I try to cling to Lizzie's hope but really, I don't know what to think.

July 2012, the long walk of shame down to Urogynaecology

I think of language as I walk deep into the bowels of a sparkling new building.

As I am about to find out, Urogynaecology is a new landscape. Weirder than *Green Wing* and less sexy than *Grey's Anatomy* – all wipe-clean surfaces, and machines that give you a printout of how much, and how fast, you've weed.

Given what is happening behind the oak-look fire doors, the department is impersonal and nondescript and I feel a bit giddy and tearful. I want my now grown-up sisters, and my mum. My women to remind me I am not about to disappear. What I really don't want to do is remove my knickers.

And I'm still not sure how to talk about my privates. In Shakespeare's time 'nothing' was a synonym for women's parts – literally 'no thing', an absence of a willy. I'm about to show my nothing to loads of people I have never met. People who work as a team and all know each other. Have found and assessed each other's comfort zones. I wonder, once they've seen my nothing, will any of these people think they know me? I have a list of questions I want to ask at the end of this assessment. I cribbed them from a medical website. They are medical and sensible and about the future. But what I am still stuck on wanting to shout is:

Who are YOU though? What are you like? Would this be easier if we had a relationship? Is everyone who comes here as lost as me? And how can I be honest with you when these things make me want to cry with even my closest friends?

I disinfect my hands for the third time with ice-cold gel and wig out as the weight of it all starts to get to me. I don't want to fucking be here. I have missed out on so many things because of appointments, or ringing up and chasing them, and the endless rounds of health admin.

This room is too bright. The reception staff are too nice. It is all too clean and glowy. I feel like I will ruin the place with my sadness. My shame has bubbled to the surface; it is paint in the sun. I've come so far and got so dirty in the process, and I should run away. There's nothing to complain about really. I'm not dying, after all. I just smell and don't feel like myself.

They call my name.

'My' surgeon, a small, lithe, optimistic man who I immediately christen the Waz Wizard, takes a personal medical history. My periods, which seem to have become inexplicably heavier since childbirth, not easier as I'd hoped, my births, medication, hospital visits, continence, 'normal' bowel and bladder habits, the lot. This is a key part of being a patient, something you have to learn to do properly. You need to ensure you give your doctors all the right information for them to help you get what you need. It helps if you know what you need.

I am used to, but not 'down with', the medical history as a concept by now. I find it repetitive and boring, and slightly irritating as they have a massive paper folder on their desk, which presumably has all of this written out with the right medical terms anyway. The health tale I have to tell wrong-foots me. Even though I am the protagonist, I can't get my piss-story straight. The Waz Wizard asks how I think he can help me.

I freeze. I don't know which treatment would be right for me.

He asks me why I am here, how I've been. I know why he has done that, but I still duck into a tailspin. Defensive, apologetic, nervy. Every time I try to say something, like 'I know I wet myself every day because my pads get wet', I feel stupid. When I tell him it is worse when I am on my period, I panic. Perhaps everyone wees themselves when they're on their period. Maybe it said that on the Tampax leaflet and I have just forgotten. I start trying to think if there has been a day recently when I didn't soak a pad running up the stairs. Perhaps I should just cross my legs. Shhh.

Suddenly feeling a bit scared all the time feels small fry too. Who am I to imagine that my fanny is so special that I should be treated like royalty? Maybe all women put up with this and they are just too polite to say so and I've spent years making mountains (of Tena Lady) from molehills of shame.

I try really, really hard to concentrate, but I muddle up which birth injury goes with which son.

All the while, the doctor listens carefully and takes notes. He looks sorry, but not involved, when my voice goes high and *mywordsruntogetherbreathlessly*. He lets a nurse with a deep throaty laugh coax out the story with 'mmms' and 'ahs'. Let's call her Carol, she has a Carol sort of face and almost makes me feel safe. I feel like a five-year-old writhing at the dentist, or a woman on a bridge being talked down. I half expect them to give me a sticker at the end, or section me.

An entire area of study, the Medical Humanities, now exists with a focus on ideas like 'medical narrative', the story of us and our illness and treatment. It is something patients can own and it can help recovery. I study this online, learning about children with terminal cancer and how hard the idea of a story is for their parents and carers, as it forces them to think about the ending, death, which the child itself usually knows is coming. I read about clinics where patients work with artists or storytellers to build body stories, finding meaning in the narrative of recovery.

I'm scared that the narrative of me might forever be broken, that my medical history is now incoherent and unreliable. As I fumble for dates and words, what I offer is poetry not reportage, a deranged conflation – medical terms and interjections, most of the right notes but none of them in the right order. The story I'm telling is mine, but it's horrible. It's repetitive and familiar because I spend my life daring myself to pass it off as jokes, and then writing about it on the Internet to pretend that by the chutz-pah of self-publication I don't need the bit where I think about it and process it properly.

But I do need that to happen. I do need to own it.

The surgeon is convinced regardless of my wavering. He only loses his confident bounce when I blurt something about hoping he doesn't think I'm wasting his time and he stares straight at me like I am speaking a different language.

He deals with pissy knickers all day long and he's INCREDULOUS that I am putting up with this. His eyes pop out of his head when I say how long I persevered with Lizzie in my second round of physio.

I can see the problem. I am cynical, strung out, and tired. I don't find the simplicity of his view, or his sincerity, easy to under-stand. Even my fem-rage has deflated somewhere in the mess. A flat offer to try and help as quickly as possible feels obscene and dangerous, like a scam. Their forward motion and earnestness, their commitment to 'sorting stuff out', feels odd and wrong after so much fumbling around. I have accepted every useless message about incontinence fed to me my entire life. I wasn't expecting them to think it is important, very important in fact, to fix me and all the other women in the waiting room.

He writes to my GP describing my urinary incontinence as 'florid' and organises scans to assess what surgical options will be best. He also books me in for an imaging investigation called Urodynamics. 'At least that sounds jolly,' I think.

That night, I blog about the appointment and my nerves, fears and shame. I have an extraordinary response. Women I know well, and women I don't know at all, contact me. Many are going through similar things but feeling alone. Some say I am articulating the things they can't voice outside their own heads. Sharing makes me feel good, but comes at a price. Now everyone knows how I feel.

Also, the surgeon had surprised me most, not with his intensely mechanical examination, which involves inserting a speculum, asking me to raise a leg up like a synchronised swimmer and then telling me to bear down, but by saying: 'You've been unwell for a long time now, Luce.'

October 2012, imaging department, somewhere medical underground

As soon as I get my letter about my urodynamics, I'm intrigued. How can they see my bladder filling without cutting me open? I'm not sure. But I can tell there will be an element of performance to it. 'Perhaps it will be like Pussy Riot, but without the balaclavas,' I think. I will be an actual piss artist. Ha.

'This is D-Day, Luce,' I say to myself, as I arrive. 'The public analysis of your twice-broken twat.' It feels momentous. The big assessment to check whether surgery is an option.

Everyone is very kind and upbeat. We meet the incontinence nurse from my first appointment again, Carol. Her straight-up kindness is so quietly but firmly reassuring that she makes all the catheters and things just seem, well, normal. Honestly, at one point later she's fiddling with my arse to add a probe to monitor my strength (I think), a probe that tickles mildly like the other wires that seem to be attaching me to a machine, and she manages it all with the air of a kindly school nurse giving me a pad after I've started my period in PE.

But before that, before we can get to the really fun stuff, I enter a surreal nightmare of David Lynch style proportions. We really are in the bowels of the hospital now, in the sinister world of the special toilets.

Being on the edge of help brings into relief just how appalling and upsetting being incontinent has been. And how fucking lonely too. But at least today I won't piss on my clothes, because a nurse has just asked me to take them all off! I act cool and huddle with my husband in a cubicle. He's here, along with a pair of lucky socks, for moral support.

'It's going to be all right, isn't it?' I whisper to him. 'What if I make a mess of it?'

'This is why we're here,' he says, ruefully, and kisses me on the nose. We have the letter and we've turned up at the right time with my bladder full, as asked. We've done our bit. And he's right: this is why we are here. I calm down. The test might be a bit embarrassing, but I'm ready. I'm an old-hat at humiliation, after all.

'That's lovely,' says Carol, when I emerge in my two hospital gowns, one covering my front, the other on backwards for hiding my bottom. 'But you'd better take your socks off, my love.'

I nearly laugh. And die. She sends me to the toilet. Adding in passing, 'Use the one with the silver seat, not the normal one.'

I think, '*If you sprinkle when you tinkle, please be neat and wipe the seat.*'

'I can do toilets,' I think as I enter the test room. 'I can sit on the silver bog like the queen.' I look down. There's a propeller at the bottom of the silver toilet's bowl. A propeller! I have to sit and wee onto a spinning propeller. I wonder if this will be the best bit.

I'm standing on a threshold, surveying both loos. My bum is cold in my gowns. I take a deep breath. I can wee on a propeller, I'm a grown-up. I sit on the silver loo and try to 'relax'. No dice. The wall moves. There is a hidden door. Though I've locked the main door to the corridor where my husband is sitting with all my clothes in a plastic bag, the room is somehow connected to some other rooms behind it. And there is Carol! She's popped up, from behind me, to see how I'm doing. She turns on a tap to help.

Spurred on by running water, I wee and Carol checks the readout before ushering me to another room, where I am to be fastened to the monitors. She whispers good luck and asks me to lie on a big wipe-clean bed, attaching a technically named straw which they will later use to fill my bladder 'to capacity'.

I'm scared and intrigued. We're in a radiography room now, and some people are milling around. Carol checks nothing she's inserted is catching on anything. Everything looks bleached out in the unkind lighting. The staff are in those anti-radioactive anti-X-ray aprons. They look to me like they are in galoshes.

It is not unlike the bit in *Charlie and the Chocolate Factory* where they enter the bright, white Wonka TV studio and Mike Teavee shrinks himself, except Mr Wonka didn't look at Mike Teavee's urethra. I feel very small though.

'Don't worry, Luce, this is a wet room,' says Carol.

'You mustn't be embarrassed if you leak on the floor or anywhere,' the radiographer concurs. 'This is why you are here.'

The set-up is pretty weird. I have wires and tubes protruding from all manner of holes once I've been plugged in. I'm feeling a bit strange and pale. But now I'm hooked-up, half woman half machine, there are some new people arriving. The room is getting crowded, full of people ready to watch somebody fill my bladder up bit by bit. They've explained it very carefully but I don't really understand – they've just made me empty my bladder all out. I wonder who is going to do the filling.

'This is Jim the scientist,' says Carol. (At least he looks like a Jim.)

'Awesome!' I think.

'And there's your consultant, Mr Waz Wizard.' (Although obviously she doesn't call him that.)

I feel rude. I want to sit up and acknowledge them both, but I don't want to move on the bed in case I dislodge something.

Jim the scientist is very kind and manages to be discreet while talking loudly and clearly about a series of fictional scenarios that may or may not chime with how much I need a wee, as somebody (Carol?) pumps cold stuff through a catheter up what I think is my urethra. It is chilly, but Jim has questions.

He keeps asking me, as my bladder fills, if I feel like I need or want to do a pee.

The hilarious thing is that though I can see, with my eyes, that my bladder is growing, and though I feel really bloody odd, I don't know. I don't know if I need a wee. Or want one, for that matter. For the first time in five years of being ruled by my bladder and hyperconscious of its failing, I have no idea.

'I don't know,' I murmur on repeat.

'Would you pop to the toilet now?' he asks, keeping it real. 'Would you go in if you walked past a loo right now? Are you beginning to feel any pressure?'

'I am feeling the pressure, Jim,' I think. 'But on the "would you nip for a pee?" question I have no idea.'

I don't know why. Nerves? Worry? Shame? Yes, probably shame.

They assure me there is no right answer – I don't manage to joke about how that isn't the sort of test I like. I hate tests with no right answer, where I can't get an A*. Though I do crack them up when Carol asks if I'm allergic to anything and I say, 'Cats' (true).

'I left mine at home today,' says nice, nice Carol with a wink.

'Good job,' I say out loud in the way you never actually do. 'NOBODY wants me to sneeze.'

They laugh politely. I can make the wet room work, I decide. This is all material.

And then they tip the bed until I am standing. I rise like Hannibal Lecter and see all the people (who are so nice), the people who have come to watch how and why and when and how much I leak.

The very nice radiologist is soothing throughout and warns me I might feel faint; some people do apparently. I feel like I'm dying, again. But I hold my nerve and am shaken into reality when I realise I actually do really, really need the loo now my bladder is full and I am standing up. There are five or six people in the room. I can't count or be that accurate because I feel like I've had four glasses of warm white wine and no dinner. I'm here for this, I womanned up, but I still nearly cry, nearly cry like a little girl in the supermarket who knows she's about to wet her big girl pants.

The next bit is even worse. They don't let you go once you are desperate. Oh no. You have to cough and move so they can see what bits of you don't work. To help, because I am helpful, I agree to lift my gown so they can get all views. A fucked-up Marilyn Monroe on the grate. A crazed can-can girl with my skirt pulled up. I wonder if I can cover my face with the gown, but that seems melodramatic so I just hold it up above my groin.

Still, I fathom, I get to watch my bladder moving and empty-ing on a luminous screen as I cough and they see a slosh of my urine hit the floor. This detail, showing my bladder's failure on a big screen, almost convinces me that my incontinence isn't some-thing I've made up completely. I do start wishing I'd shaved my legs though.

Then comes the finale. I'm standing, with spurts of wee escaping, depending on what I'm asked to do. I'm trying hard not to be nervous as I've read somewhere that could affect the test(!).

But then they ask if I would be able to empty my bladder completely, right there, in front of them all.

Time stops.

I'm like 'Now? Here? Doing a massive wee on my feet? *Being watched?*'

I emit a squeak.

'Don't worry,' says the nice radiographer.

'You don't have to. Some women find it too embarrassing,' says Carol.

'It would help,' says the consultant, 'but there's no pressure.' The room expects, though.

And I'm still thinking 'SOME? Only SOME of them find it too embarrassing? Not ALL? Jesus, I'm far less cool about this than I thought.'

They seemed a little surprised at how upset I look, though I possibly imagined that as my head is all buzzy and light.

'Deep breaths,' I think. 'If we're being realistic AT LEAST TWO OF THE ADULTS IN THIS ROOM HAVE STUCK THEIR FINGER UP MY BUM BEFORE. And be reasonable, the rest have been so reassuring and respectfully upbeat. And, bonus, they keep telling you you're doing really, really well.'

I decide to ride it out with a deep breath and just, well, stand and wee everything left in my bladder everywhere. So I say, in a slightly scared little voice:

'Um, okay …'

I take a breath, with a shocked but defeated expression. The radiographer and Carol suddenly understand my abject misery. They fly over and save me from the most humiliating thing of all time.

'No, no, my love,' says one. 'You don't have to just wee on your feet!'

'He means will you wee into this machine here?' confirms the other. I am saved.

They hand me a she-wee attached to something that looks so oddly mechanical and homemade, it resembles a prop from *Chitty Chitty Bang Bang*. It is to measure my flow. I get top marks. Go me! I am allowed to leave and get my clothes back on.

The day isn't over. When I'm a bit sticky but no longer naked from the waist down we reconvene. We have a long meeting, a detailed discussion, another, clothes off again, examination from the surgeon as he checks for my prolapse, during which I urinate freely like a tacky European fountain. But I am high on humiliation by now. The Waz Wizard leaves the room so I can sort myself out but Carol stays. She even helps me wipe my ankles when my legs start shaking and won't stop.

'He's here to help you,' she says of the surgeon, who is sprightly but assured and even more Mr Wonka-ish now he isn't in a weird lead suit. I love Carol and the surgeon now. They have a quiet but enthusiastic calm and confidence. Perhaps because they actually spend their days making life less shit for people and mending stuff.

I still almost fuck it all up by wittering. And in the time it takes for me to put my clothes back on a second time, I have convinced myself the consultant is going to tell me that he won't or can't help me because I'm too young, or I haven't done enough pelvic floor exercises, or I don't deserve it, that I'm just whinging, or I'm too fat, or … something.

He humours me for a bit and then pulls a face and describes my stress incontinence as 'off the scale'.

Good or bad? I want to know, but he beats me to it. He can tell it is awful.

'What do you want to do?' he asks, and boom, finally the feminist in me wakes up again. She roars to raise the dead.

'I want you to do an operation and stop this now, please, because I can't bear it any more,' she says.

And that's what he offers – to try and fix me with an operation called a colposuspension whenever he can next fit me in. Then he thanks me for coming, which is pretty nice of him given I have just pissed all over the wall of his office. For shame.

Chapter 15

History

I may be seeing her less but I am still very perplexed by Lizzie's idea that I am a woman *in trouble* and that other people can see I need help. It is true that I am in a fix. But any anger or fire I feel at my lot is pissed on with a tidal wave of guilt. Deep down, I have a keen sense that I'm a social burden wasting endless time and resources with my poor pelvic floor and poorer efforts. People, medical and not, say 'no no no' when I voice this. But I fervently believe it is true.

I decide to look into the history of my condition and particular brand of being in trouble – have women always felt their fanny concerns were something they should be ashamed of fighting for, or is it just me?

One thing I find is that gynae-broken women – my tribe – are generally expected to sort themselves out, ideally quietly and out of public view.

You can see it in the trajectory of female physicians – those who broke the mould or broke new ground. Elizabeth Garrett Anderson is a prime example. Despite repeated rejections by male institutions and having to travel widely to collect (and repeat) qualifications, Garrett Anderson was the first woman to qualify as a doctor in Britain (and the first woman to be elected a mayor!). She was also a wife, a mother, a dean and the founder of the New Hospital for Women in London, a place where all the staff and patients were women. According to the Science Museum, Garrett

Anderson, daughter of a pawnbroker, was inspired to take up medicine after meeting Dr. Elizabeth Blackwell – the first female MD to qualify from a US medical school in 1849, who set up the New York Infirmary for Women and Children. When Garrett Anderson became dean of the London School of Medicine for Women, she brought Blackwell to the UK to make her head of Gynaecology, and set about campaigning for a new Act of Parliament to be passed in 1876, which would allow women to qualify in medicine.

Yes, there was no doubt an historical element of squeamishness, propriety and modesty to early female doctors specialising in women's issues, but it masks a deeper problem that exists the world over to this day. Women's health is a problem for women to solve, like the experience of over half the global population is a curio, a special interest. And as if a person having children has no impact on men, who have no links to the process – are not, for example, created by it in the first place, or instrumental in its perpetuation.

In the eighteenth century The City Of London Lying-in Hospital opened for the wives of tradesmen suffering the 'terrors, pains and hazards of child-birth'. Women *in particular* were encouraged to donate money to run it. Though only caring for married women of 'good character', as was common, the place interested me as even back then the issue of birth-damaged women and their inability to function is right there in the hospital's founding literature. Post-partum problems, both social and personal, were clearly understood to be frequent. And that includes damage from delivery in general, not just catastrophic births, which were presumably common in a time before decent analgesia, anaesthetic, infection control, or midwifery practices.

'It cannot but greatly move our Compassion to reflect how many unhappy Women even after a safe Delivery, for want of proper Diet, Medicines and Attendance, [have] either perished, or

been deprived of the Use of their Limbs, or otherwise impaired in their Constitutions, so as to become useless to their Families and burdensome to the Public.'

The more I read, the more I realise that I stand at the end of a long line of women whose birth didn't kill them but did leave them reliant on help. Thanks to modern medicine and pharmaceutical invention, plus the massive luck of geography and economics, I have access to help to manage my problems. But I wonder how many incontinent or PND-ish women in the twenty-first century would still be contained in this neat burdensome euphemism of 'impaired' constitution.

Even if I don't let my depression talk, objectively I am a drain on resources. All incontinent people are. All the drugs I've taken. All the space my condition takes up in my brain, hindering productive thoughts. Not to mention the environmental waste. Pads and fake knickers and clothes thrown away. All the extra washing. It's easy to absorb guilt. I am very prone to it.

It riles me that, despite our excellent healthcare from the NHS, I foot a considerable bill just to keep my life in motion. And the cost to the individual patient is a real issue. But as well as being another disadvantage for people with disabilities and chronic conditions, perhaps this also contributes to the lack of impetus, or a broader conversation about what we can do to improve continence care across the board. There is a bigger story at play too – patients may be coughing up a lot, but countries could save squillions if they had a more concerted and forward-thinking attitude to preventing and curing continence problems.

Countless studies explore the economic impact of incontinence, which makes me wonder: why aren't policymakers and politicians more vocal and exercised about stopping people leaking, if only on the grounds of saving money?

The Continence Foundation of Australia audited the socio-economic cost of incontinence especially for geriatric patients (a large proportion of incontinent patients), drilling down to the spend on laundry, care for the bedridden and homebound, nappies, care homes. Women are over-represented in the groups of both patient and carer, so bear a bigger cost, of course they do. It noted welfare payments, reduced productivity (and taxable income), from those unwell and giving informal care (unpaid family, neighbours), and the deadweight administration costs in health and social care. It totted up the bills for additional health problems too – from injuries rushing to the loo, infections and bedsores to mental health breakdowns, post-op complications, and the secondary price of diseases of inaction in a group more prone to diabetes and heart disease because they are afraid or unable to move.

Incontinence soaks through the fabric of society; social isolation carries financial implications, as does marriage/relationship breakdown (from incontinence and related issues in sexual function for men and women); not to mention the cost of otherwise healthy workers leaving jobs or losing their jobs due to toilet issues. Call centre staff, for example, can be reprimanded or even lose their jobs if urinary frequency is an issue for them and they have to take extra toilet breaks.

They concluded that the cost of incontinence ran into billions.

And there's more. Consider the massive cost to the environment of plastic-based products and aids, both prescribed and used at home for self-care.

Activists here in the UK now argue that it would be cheaper to invest money up front for all patients, assessing women post-birth, and then when they are menopausal, and encouraging prostate health and pelvic floor exercises in everyone. That doing this *as routine* would help break down the wall of silence and nip problems in the bud before they are entrenched. But it still falls at the same hurdle – when nobody finds a way to start a serious conversation with *everyone* about incontinence, then the cycle continues.

The history of the surgery that the Waz Wizard suggests for me also provokes thought. It is the keyhole update of a procedure called the Burch colposuspension. Complex and scary though the whole thing sounds, it seems to involve sewing my bladder more firmly in place. He recommends it confidently, partly as I am particularly young for my degree of laxity. I feel I should find out more and assess the risks myself though. They seem to range wildly, from the surgery not working at all to needing a wee bag, to bladder infections or further operations.

The op dates back to 1961, though it was amended to reduce tension in 1976, the year before I was born. For decades, it was the stress incontinence surgery gold standard. It had quite good results, but dropped out of favour in the 2000s after the emergence of mesh-based operations. These mesh ops were welcomed initially, as they were less invasive and seemed to have better short-term success rates.

In the 'TVT' operation a mesh is implanted to hold things back into place. It acts like a hammock or sling and is less invasive than the colposuspension, though neither leaves huge external scars. I want one and know people who are evangelical about this surgery.

I am jealous of the women who are offered the tension-free vaginal tape (TVT) mesh operation. It is so demoralising to find that my stupid body makes me the wrong sort of candidate. Why can't I ever fit in the 'normal' mould? I wonder. In retrospect I realise I probably had a lucky escape.

Unfortunately, over my incontinence years the potential risks and complications following the TVT op emerge, most notably in some cases that the mesh itself can disintegrate or travel around the body, tearing into other organs – and causing lasting damage and injury. Also, when this happens it can be difficult or impossible to untangle the mess. Mesh isn't always easy to remove. You can be left with fragments or whole pieces inside you, even after surgeons have attempted to get it all out. The mesh implant going

TVT Mesh and Colposuspension

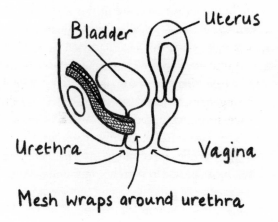

Mesh wraps around urethra

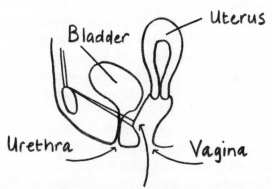

Cord lifts front vaginal wall forwards

wrong can lead to impaired mobility, chronic leg, pelvic and groin pain, UTIs and damage to nerves and nearby organs as the mesh penetrates or perforates the internal tissue. In some women, the operation can also make the vagina incredibly painful, and sex uncomfortable or even intolerable.

Though there are people for whom it appears to have worked well, campaigners have compared the use of mesh for these operations to the Thalidomide scandal in the 1960s, and meanwhile the editor-in-chief at the *BMJ* called the mesh story a 'shameful episode', riddled with injustice, pain and the silencing of patients. It is also characterised by a lack of proper reporting. Beyond the complications, and ignored female voices, are concerns about a lack of transparency over the efficacy and safety of the procedures itself, speculation around how safety evaluations were funded, and even poor disclosure or apparent lies told to some patients about the materials that would be inserted into their bodies, precluding informed consent.

It took the medical and research community many years to accept the experience of patients saying the operation was flawed (safety and effectiveness were first studied in 1996 – when I had to move on to surgical options in 2011, it was still the gold standard). Many women I speak to later talk about the lack of adequate information on risks or possible complications. Perhaps it was hard for a surgical community to accept that the easy op risked irreversible damage, given the history of failed and dangerous surgery to cure incontinence and prolapse. Stories like these make it look like medicine has failed. I think there's something deeper going on though.

My understanding is only from the sidelines, but from there I saw the coverage of the mesh story underscoring the stigma. Even when it floods the news, the underlying reason why so many women went under the knife at all is *totally ignored*. Why would anyone allow relatively untested materials into their girdles? Because, of course, continence issues are difficult, damaging and devastating. Reports touch on this and how a potent mix of mostly women's trust in establishment and doctors, feeling they couldn't say no and poor communication of risk from medics, affected patients. But very few dare to look at the dirty truth, the effect of stigma and the way people feel and are made to feel when they suffer from incontinence and how it is so awful they will often do anything to hide it: end a relationship, retreat in discomfort, lie, self-medicate, have treatment in secret, stop exercising, withdraw from society, or get chopped up.

The stigma casts a swooping shadow over the whole mesh story, with its usual stubborn recklessness. It sticks to the women as if they deserve blame for risking everything because of a trifle, when in truth, they had a condition so shameful, irritating and upsetting to their everyday life that it was unbearable. It details their pain and suffering but rarely talks about what drove women to have the operation, how incontinence also affected their lives, often catastrophically. The complications following mesh surgery have even been cited as one of the underlying causes of death, including the patient Eileen Baxter, who died in Edinburgh in 2016.

It feels a gruesome shame that incontinence can reach top billing while being simultaneously muted once again. That lives have been ruined, and the taboo has been reinforced and the situation still remains a bloody mess the world over. Even research into how and why mesh breaks down or what could be done to stop that happening is hampered by the fact that many bits of fragmented and broken mesh can't be examined in research because they are evidence in future lawsuits.

There is another social complication too – throughout the mesh surgery's complex history, women's reports of their own health complaints do not always seem to have been taken seriously, and/or what affects them, such as complications to do with painful sex, was not necessarily considered important. Many mesh campaigners complain that they were asked whether they were leak-free but not about pain, resulting in parameters of 'success' that didn't allow for the operation to be properly assessed. If a patient was dry post-op, the operation may have been chalked up as a success, with no reference to even serious complications. This said, the amount of time mesh disintegration can take to surface means it has been genuinely complicated to assess the risks.

Another line of thought I hear expressed is a horrible suspicion that the problems some women expressed about sexual function fell on unsympathetic ears until another narrative emerged, in which men became the victim. Of those women whose mesh had perforated their vagina, some had injured their male partner's penis during (often painful) sex. There's the rub: a grated penis is more of a catalyst for outrage than a woman in a wheelchair, or such intense chronic pain that she is no longer fit enough to work.

Campaigners have also focused on the influence of manufacturers and criticised the roll out of a technique with insufficient testing or information about risk.

A doctor I meet via twitter, Louise, a British GP who was forced into early retirement due to post-mesh op pain and complications, sums up the misogyny of silencing women in a blistering open letter to her former medical colleagues:

> *I do not believe there was a dark money conspiracy to implant these devices by you, but you do have a dangerously positive bias on your successes, and yes I do accept for the majority it is a successful procedure. I do however believe there is a huge unconscious negative bias among you all towards middle-aged females in chronic pain. As more information is now coming out about the risks, some of you are still choosing to downplay or actually disbelieve these facts. I do believe there was aggressive marketing and suppression of concerns by the manufacturers. I don't believe we were honestly, fully and accurately consented.*

These are feminist problems. If not being able to make informed decisions about what is placed in your fanny is not a feminist issue, I don't know what is.

And if some women's voices are not considered autonomous and important when they are describing their own pain and experiences then the landscape is broken and needs to change.

Clinicians are now working on developing Patient Decision Aids (PDAs), to ensure that shared decision-making and informed consent are assessable in Urogynaecology and Female Urology along with safety and efficacy of procedures. PDAs include worksheets with questions and boxes to fill in so patients can consider all their options and there is proof that they have been able to assess different risks and benefits. It seems strange that such simple things have not always been a part of standard best practice.

As the mesh story continues, I can only hope truth and help will continue to prevail, along with better ways of discussing risk with patients, especially for surgeries involving implants, as this would benefit all of us.

But the mesh incident isn't an isolated one. Consent looms large in the history of procedures to correct birth injuries, especially when you move beyond the lady doctors of the late Victorian era (at least until we get to Dr Arnold Kegel and his machines and dedication to reducing surgeries).

Take James Marion Sims, who invented one form of the speculum, and is often called 'the father of gynaecology'. He solved the problem of vaginal fistula, a gruesome birth injury that causes women to leak urine and faeces out of their vagina through an abnormal hole between their pelvic organs (often the rectum and vagina).

But he achieved this by performing experimental operations on women of colour kept as slaves, finessing his technique on these women after consent had been granted by their 'owners'. Sims claimed his patients clamoured to get to his one-stop fanny-chopping shop but their 'choices' – live with fistula or accept sometimes non-anaesthetised radical surgery – define powerlessness. It's an early recorded example of the medical mistreatment of black women, especially in obstetric medicine, whose 'care' was defined by racist mythology, notably the notion that black women do not feel as much pain as white women. These ideologies combine with racial bias and social factors to

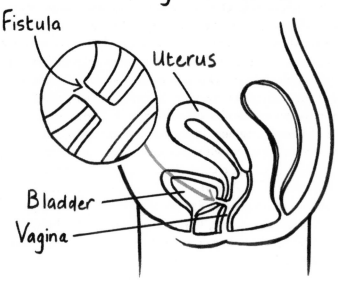

Vesicovaginal Fistula

Fistula

Uterus

Bladder

Vagina

continue to pose a threat – black mothers are still more likely to die in childbirth than white women in the UK, and the US, for example.

Their stories are not mine to tell, but I feel at least comforted that the names of the first three patient pioneers who Sims stitched up with his silver thread are now in the public domain: Lucy, Anarcha and Betsey. These are the grandmothers of urogynae surgery survivors and there have been campaigns to replace a statue of Sims in Central Park, New York, with a monument to these women instead. We all owe them a great debt.

It seems a tiresome outrage that we are still fumbling around to try and sort this out when incontinence has been a dire problem since year dot. But bladder surgery has always been fraught with danger. Many cultures and eras have ingenious contraptions, including catheters fashioned from quills, precious metal or reeds, most of which look both incredibly crude, and not that different from their sterile replacements today.

The Hippocratic Oath (which is associated with medicine even if doctors don't take it anymore) is even claimed by some scholars to include a warning about the difficulties of urological surgery – telling physicians not to cut out bladder stones, even though they are awful, as it is a specialist skill requiring a surgeon. The risks are high, slicing into the peeing places. Before he became a diarist and buried his cheese in the Great Fire of London, Samuel Pepys had a bladder stone the size of a billiard ball cut out with no anaesthetic. For his op, in 1658, he was strapped to a chair to stop him moving and screaming. Quite unusually, he survived without complications. He kept the stone as a trophy and liked to show it to visitors apparently, partly to grim them out, I'm sure, but also to celebrate wildly his escape from continence woes. I wonder what trophy my op will leave me.

Chapter 16

Surgery

Once I bit the bullet, having an op seemed like a real break-through. A relief, even. So much so that, though I looked at the risks, I didn't really explore the recovery. It was too seductive to believe it was going to be my salvation and reward, a symbolic set of closing stitches.

I knew it might be hard, but I was wrong-footed by the physical and psychological shock of stepping neatly from the world of the well to the world of the properly sick in the space of one morning. The slide from healthy but broken to poorly but possibly fixed. Barely passing GO, definitely not collecting £200.

I rocked up in a taxi, still drafting emails for work and reading *Wolf Hall*, and left three days later, drugged up, bruised, with a catheter taped to the inside of my leg, unable to speak a sentence or to read the other book I'd brought with me, *Fifty Shades of Grey*.

In my defence, it is unreadable. And also, when I went in, I was already half-crazy from all the years of slow-motion physio, chafed thighs and performing the 'sneeze and soak' every time I had the temerity to spray any perfume. (Half a decade of needing two outfits for any event.)

That's not to mention a seemingly endless string of urinary infections, which meant antibiotics (and their wicked sister side-kick, perma-thrush). The trouble with endless, low-rent, *not that 'serious'* health problems is that they make your brain ache with the mundanity of discomfort.

Talking of my brain, it had also started to sort of ebb away from me again. It wasn't the prospect of a quite invasive old-fashioned operation, which was my surgeon's clear recommendation, that finally broke me. It was that I had to keep telling people about it in a sensible sober voice, often face-to-face. Disclosing the operation's name meant letting people know what a mess I had been in, and for how long. And that became perhaps the biggest challenge yet. There's something very daunting about parading your pubic brokenness in public, especially when you still feel your condition is a direct result of an inadequacy in you. It would have been easier if I'd invented a less mortifying procedure, like having my sweat glands polished, a lightbulb removed from my arse, or extensive treatment for long-term genital warts.

I put myself under aggressive pressure to tell the whole truth, even though perhaps at that point I wasn't ready. I forced myself to explain to HR the true nature of the appointments, going beyond euphemisms like 'women's stuff' and using proper medical terms. I even stopped scribbling out clinic names on my letters. It was hard to own up to the type of broken I was. I suppose I could have lied, but it felt wrong to perpetuate the stigma if by night I was still ranting online about how important it was for people to stop the silence.

Speaking frankly in the open, with '*normal*', continent people was hard. Hard to know how to get the point across before anyone was too kind, or with the best of intentions suggested yoga, or said I was like their nan. I'm glad I did though. It paved the way for building a healthier, more self-protective brand of honesty later.

I'd had two operations before – one to fix my fractured elbow, the other to remove a cyst in my eye – so *clearly* I was an expert patient who could handle this laparoscopic fandangle, and I felt confident, blasé even.

Blasé was only surface-deep though; part of my subconscious brain was scared. I started writing letters to my children 'just in case' and rearranging the kitchen shelves to *Livingetc* standards.

The night before I went in, I even painted one of the spindles on my banister red. A stripe of terror in a world of grey. I know. MAD.

But still. I was pretty sure we'd thought of everything by asking one of my little sisters to come down and stay, armed with glossy magazines, new pyjamas, Haribo and dried fruit (to keep me regular).

11 February 2013, large teaching hospital, 6 a.m.

We trundle in super early and I take an Instagram shot of the looming skyline as we drive into town, tall buildings gleaming like proud wands in the biting February dawn, good luck charms for my magic cure.

Though such fancies can't distract me from a new pressing concern: I have just started my period. I can't tell if it will be a problem for a lady-part op.

The Waz Wizard is unperturbed by a bit of menstrual blood. He's in his natural habitat, the eerie bright surgery wards, and he's super-motivated about getting cracking on my bladder. He's even brought a friend with him! Another wee doctor. As we run through the paperwork, he repeats his kindly offer to stick a coil in while they are in there, having remembered my heavy periods and my feeling that I get more depressed around my cycle. A Mirena coil, he says, might make my periods lighter and me happier. I think: *In for a penny.*

He wants to tell me what they are going to do, and how, with diagrams. This is quite confusing when you haven't eaten for hours as instructed and suddenly remember why people are scared of operations.

The Waz Wizard does a little drawing of my bladder-neck and the entry points either side of my belly and then asks me to sign another form saying I know the risks. I have forgotten the risks. I understood them last week. But Christ, I'm still struggling to say 'laparoscopic colposuspension' without feeling like a dick.

Laparoscopic Surgery

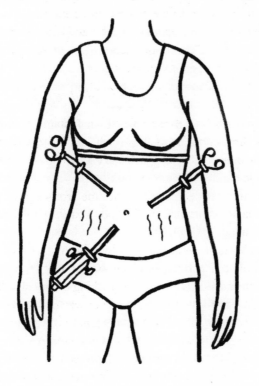

I just about pay attention as he summarises them again patiently, adding that they are going in near my belly button.

'Oh God,' I think. 'They are going to be staring at my tummy. How humiliating.'

I double-check my overnight bag. Roll-top soft pyjama bottoms with wide legs, soft bras and vests I can sleep in, a nice cardigan that goes below my bottom for warmth, and two nighties in case the temporary wee bag doesn't fit under the PJs. None of these match the green hold-up style compression stockings, which make me feel like a whore in a 1950s Western.

'Yee-haw,' I think, toying with embracing this look for the rest of my life. I still might.

And then they are gone. To check everyone else in, and put us in a running order. I keep reading my novel, trying not to imagine my stretch-marked blancmange belly with a camera skewered through it, as people check my blood pressure and ask the same questions again and again.

I'm with my husband; my sister has stayed to breakfast the children and will meet me when I wake up. We've nailed it on the organisation front. Nerves are jangling though and I still can't help but answer 'cats' every time I'm asked if I'm allergic to anything.

It is only when I see the last doctor, an anaesthetist doing his final checks, that I see someone has handwritten CATS on my wristband.

'What is CRTS?' he asks, looking frantically at my notes after misreading the paper bracelet. 'Is it a medication you are allergic to?'

We laugh, how we laugh, and I pee down my legs. I can feel the smudge of that and period blood between my thighs as I've had to take my tampon out. I wish I'd lost more weight beforehand, but there's not time now. A door opens and look! It's the lovely Carol again. She's here! I am beyond relieved. She's helped many women take these steps, in a corridor that feels and looks a lot like a space station. She's made it okay for them. I resist the urge to hold her hand tight. We turn a corner to a new room. It's almost a thrill: it's called a theatre after all. My audience awaits.

Because I am ambulatory and unsick, I walk right into the room where they will put me to sleep, see the military-looking trolley and have to climb onto it. I'm laying myself out like a Christmas turkey. I'm meat on a plate. They say something about how they may transfer me again, but I'm not sure to what; the minute people start moving my body around for me, I begin to lose track of where I am. That's how quick it is: one minute a living, walking, joke-cracking, free-widdling person, only slightly stressed; the next, gone, a thing, a slab, having to grasp at my buzzing thoughts juddering up towards the lights like bluebottles – ugly, intrusive, out of place in this sterile space.

I get it in my head that I shouldn't move at all in case they can't find the right bit of me to cut up. I don't like to think they will probably move me around endlessly once I'm under. But it's okay: it's like a reunion. Or a flashback in an '80s soap opera. It's Bouncer's dream. Suddenly, everyone from urodynamics is here again for a party in my bladder – and I'm looking up at their faces, their matching uniforms, clean and pressed and about to be spattered in person blood. And I think I can see the operating theatre beyond the doors. I'm starting to imagine them watching my innards on their little TV. Do they go through the belly button because there's some magic umbilical tunnel I never realised was still there, or to minimise scarring? I don't know.

I forget to ask because: *Look!* There's the nice anaesthetist again, leaning over and looking at my face to signal he's ready to start. He's so keen that it seems churlish to ask a question. They are raring to go.

Carol winks at me and squeezes my hand because she's really, really nice. Or someone does, they all have masks now. And I suspect they can all hear the quiver coming back into my voice. The anaesthetist – who, like me, is probably trying not to think of a pussy joke about the whole CATS allergy thing in a gynae-cological surgery – loses his air of newness and takes charge. He runs down his list and talks to me. He's the boss of the big drugs and checking I'm alive.

I take a deep breath. I'm going in. They ask me to count down from ten. Twice. On the second 'eight', I'm gone.

11 February 2013, later that morning

The next thing I hear is someone telling me forcefully: 'Don't panic.'

I panic. This isn't right.

I lurch to vomit and then I look around. I'm definitely in the fucking operating theatre. Shit. Still in the room. This is funky déjà-vu. My brain pulses.

I wonder if I've just had a panic attack so they've stopped the performance. If they've suddenly had a real emergency and had to delay my stupid, self-indulgent fanny op. Perhaps the anaesthetic didn't work. Or a cat walked in?

'Luce, Luce, it is over. The operation's finished,' says the familiar voice, with purpose, as if she might have said it before.

I'm scared. My lips are tingling but I think I've still got arms somewhere. One hand is sore, I think it has a cannula in. I can't feel my legs, or the meeting of my thighs. Shit ...

Is it Carol talking? And wasn't I just here? Something's different. There are pipes up my nose. And electronic sounds. I look around and try to tell Carol, 'I am still in the operating theatre,' but I can't talk as there's something in my mouth ...

Shit, I think, maybe I just drifted off between 'eight' and 'seven' and have lost track of my mind. Or, double, triple shit, I've woken up mid-surgery. Oh GOD. I am about to become one of those people who make £250 from *Take A Break*.

Or maybe I'm dead and Carol was St Peter all along ...

But here's Carol, lovely, lovely Carol again, shh-ing me kindly, or at least somebody Carol-like looming above me in a papery cap. She reassures me that I'm not dead and explains. The recovery suite is backlogged somehow so they've woken me up here in the surgery room instead. Efficient!

I drift off again.

The next time I wake, I realise why I can't talk. I have an oxygen mask on! I'm Maverick in *Top Gun*. I am feeling very trippy, but the oxygen is nice. And I don't need to make much effort to breathe, which is good because thinking is hard enough.

There's a lot of encouragement to breathe properly. I am waking and sleeping and listening to the instructions and trying really hard but drifting easily into not breathing all that much. It isn't a struggle to breathe, nor is it a struggle not to. I'm quite enjoying myself. Apparently, it is caused by all the morphine and I'm happily sacking off doing something simple, giving up. I'm not normally a slacker. I don't mean to keep drifting off. I end up backlogging the poor jam-packed recovery suite even more, as I can't be trusted to breathe in and out without a nurse telling me when to do it.

I'm not at all frightened once I know I'm alive, but I'm less happy when they ship me out to the ward and I realise that now the cocktail of drugs is wearing off, I'm really very sore. Every time I move, it feels like I'm splitting in half somehow. But I don't want to piss anyone off or waste their time for hours. So I piss them off and waste their time for a couple of days, not really articulating my own pain threshold and so getting pretty distressed and sick. Well done me.

The surgeons are marginally less chipper when they come to check up on me. But they are desperate to start talking about how it has gone – very well, apparently. The coil's also in. Bullseye. The bladder neck has been firmly sewn up now and it's less likely to wiggle. They have high hopes. Also, they seem to be saying something about my vagina and lifting it or something else up. They are using their hands to illustrate, acting out my operation like a game of charades. They seem *very* keen to tell me this.

I glare. Do they really imagine I can't tell they did *something down there?* The stretched-and-mauled-around-bruise-y sensation of my sore vagina area floods my brain. Perhaps, they seem to think, I didn't fully understand what they just said, so they mime it again for clarity. Momentarily, I forget to be helpful and groan out loud. I'm back in my first labour – I'm Regan in *The Exorcist* all over again. Which is fitting as she also had a lot of trouble with a devil in her crack.

'I think she'd like you to stop talking about that bit,' my sister explains. 'I don't think she likes it.'

Also provoking unhappiness are the drains. Horrible pipes oozing rusty fluids with floaty red bits into bags by the side of my bed to stop me swelling up. This sort of disgusting body soup is usually hidden by our skin. 'Clever old, nice old, good old skin,' I think, looking at mine, all iodine-yellow and rubbery near the entry points and scars, and promise to moisturise regularly for the rest of my days. Good old skin. Saving us from seeing this revolting stuff. I'll never moan about bruises or wrinkles or cellulite again.

The operation aftermath is awful. My sister gamely stays with me as I cry and moan on her but tell the doctors I'm fine. She's there for a long time and then goes to help with my kids so my husband can drop by too. I'm so grateful they are doing so much and I miss them all the second they turn to leave. As I stiffen against the pain on my arrangement of tubes and pillows I cry myself to sleep, quietly.

Worst of all, she's back in the middle of the night. Not my sister, sadly, but Mad Luce, with the sparky eyes shielding her ferocious, burning fear.

My recovery isn't over as quickly as the leaflet said it would be. I'm kept in an extra day on the wards. Visitors come and go and are greeted by bags of wee and my inability to chat. I have to learn how to ask for help, how to tell the truth. I am not giggling or nervous any more. I hurt. A lot.

I'm useless at estimating pain thresholds. When I say I'm not sure what they mean by 10 out of 10, the nurses explain maths to me but I don't have the heart to explain my real confusion: what comparisons are we using here? Years later, my eldest son sprains his wrist. Asked to mark his pain out of 10 he says 'TEN', emphatically, despite not looking too bothered.

'I don't think he has ever hurt any more than this,' I have to explain to the bemused registrar. 'For him, this four *is* a 10.'

It was only halfway through day two that the ward sister confirms how the system works. Noticing that I have to stop three paces from my bed for a little cry and a retch, my face a picture of terror as I realise that both the bed and the toilet are now *too far away for me to get to*, she explains it: involuntary crying with even tiny movements = 10.

See also: whimpering, vomming, howling, passing out, and holding your breath as you lean back into your pillow to brace for as long as you can, or being frozen in pain and unable to make a sound. Luckily, I was wearing my new cardigan, so I looked SMOKING HOT.

The friends stream in endlessly, armed with the fruit I requested, but I can't work out how to get better. Nobody makes me feel ashamed or seems openly revolted by me even with my urine on display – perhaps when push comes to shove, being confronted with someone we love's incontinence just shows we all have bodies; bodies that sometimes break.

One of the poor sods, Ally, ends up holding my drainage bag as I try to get out of bed.

'Is this your piss?' she asks slightly tentatively when I thrust it into her arms.

I shrug apologetically, but she just gives me her arm to help me get down.

I wish I was less exposed, it feels like ritualistic humiliation. But also, it is humbling.

Another friend arrives. They are so kind, they are taking shifts! She has to help me go to the toilet, sitting with me like a child. Luckily, I hurt too much to give a shit about anything, though I can't actually do one.

She rubs my arms. I try to remember I must tell her what a good mum she must be. Then she scours my charts and marches up to the nurses to sort the whole situation out. She's my phar-macological angel.

'You haven't given her the latest doses,' she tells them. 'And she's sobbing.' She must explain the constipation too as they start giving me sachets.

I had a nice scarf on though. Bingo. A scarf is an essential item for any situation where you are too poorly to be at home but don't wish to look like an anaemic ham with tits all over the place and a face as pale as a waxwork dummy. The scarf distracts from all of that (at least I'm pretty sure it does …) and the act of buying it feels like the sort of thing someone writing for *Goop* would do.

13 February 2013, unlucky for some, a London terrace house, on the sofa

I go home after several days. The house is full of flowers. Sneezy. My book group sends gifts: vintage literary filth by Harold Robbins, a little bell with a stag on it to ring for attention as I recline on the sofa, and a selection of lush new pants, ethically sourced, to make up for my continence product landfill. Too skimpy for pads, they're for when the operation works and I am clean again. If you ever have a friend having this type of op, these are the ideal gifts, along with readymade meals, and love.

I set up a sort of boudoir den in my lounge, hoping to recline with wraps and blankets casually draped over any scars, drink herbal tea and recover while entertaining people. In reality, I struggle to get upstairs to the loo with a disgusting sack of urine taped to my knee. And terrified of getting the tubes caught up in the duvet, I scrunch the blankets into a pile to be a ladder for my boys to climb onto me, and secretly cry to myself at night because I miss picking them up just as much as they miss me doing it. I scare them because I hug just a bit too hard and a bit too long – when, that is, I can reach the eldest, who hides himself away, terrified of the pipes and plumbing on display. I can't use the nice toiletries people have bought me either, as they would a) sting and b) require climbing into a bath, which I am pretty certain would crack me in half forever.

14 February 2013, still on the sofa

'Happy fucking Valentine's Day,' I think as I log onto Facebook. The wee bag itches and hurts. It makes me feel awful. And look horrible. My lucky, lucky husband. I am a *catch*.

I toy with trying to have a romantic meal on the living room floor but instead panic, because I still can't control the pain that well and it becomes an out-of-body experience. Romantic.

'I was fine a few days ago,' I think glumly, filled with urine and self-pity. 'FINE. I pissed myself a bit – so what? And now I've made the worst mistake ever by making myself crazy mad and sick when really, I should have just learned to cope and accept all this pishy bullshit as my prize for having babies. They're great, after all. *They're* worth it.'

Mainly, though, I am fixated on the tube. The tube that empties wee into a bag. Watching the amber liquid edging down the clear hose. I can't believe I have it taped to me. In me. It feels so oppressive, sore and precarious. I can't tell if it is infected or just supposed to feel like that, but then I am high. We end up at a doctor's in the middle of the night as I'm so ill and agitated it's hard to tell if I am disoriented by infection and drugs, or just mad as hell.

I ask if I can 'just pull the fucking thing out' but the locum won't let me. Even with her medical degrees, she'd get in trouble for that. She ups my pain meds and prescribes antibiotics the size of Cadbury Mini Eggs instead.

The next day I'm still burbling. Rocking on pain relief and so obsessed with the catheter that I stare at it wild-eyed, with ghoulish fascination as if it might come to life. Having to go home with one was presented as an unlikely possibility, not a definite. We start to wonder if the pain drugs are fuzzing my brain. I return to the GP and hand them back to her, saying they are making me mad. Her face is a picture as I place in her hands a veritable haul, packets and individual tablets, sticking together where I've held them too tightly in my sweaty hands as I sat in the waiting room. I say I think that it is best she has them.

'HAPPY THURSDAY, nice lady doctor,' I think.

She extends my sick note.

February 2013, a few days later, back at the hospital, done

My mum takes me for my post-op check. My belly is only achy, but my fanny still feels so swollen and tight that I honestly wonder if they've stitched me together completely, and that far from leaking, I'll never be able to piss again.

Carol greets us, with a student nurse and jug. They have a look at the scars ('lovely') and the catheter ('Not lovely,' I point out). Carol explains the op to the nurse, they talk about my age. They are kind but I have lost my lustre. I try to be polite but it is hard to work out how to say anything apart from, 'I feel horrible.' Or to admit I have barely pooed since before the operation and all the strong drugs. So much for apricots and Tangfastics. Everything is still sore, though the entry wounds from the skewers are already smaller than gummy bears and the bruising's fading. I feel cheated. I wanted battle scars. I am also mortified that I haven't been able to wash my feet.

Carol doesn't mind too much and confirms, as I'd begun to fear, that they had shaved some of my pubes for the op. She was clear this was standard and that they told me. I get a flashback to a Bic razor.

'You did it!' I say, jolting at the memory. She smiles. Kindly.

She removes the catheter gently and with no tugging. She's an expert but I'm wobbling afterwards and feel faint.

Then she confirms that the jug wasn't for show. I have to walk around the hospital for the rest of the day, measuring my pee until I've done a set amount, then return to the department to find them. I wonder if we'll be minutes, hours or days. But I'm free to roam, with my mother and my jug.

As we walk around, I worry I am broken and my nerve endings are shot. I can't walk that far, so we wind up camped near the disabled loos. I still need a handle or a helpful husband to help me off the bog. I feel sure everyone knows what my jug is for, but it is too big for my handbag. I eventually manage a wee on my own. It starts slow but it only stings and aches a bit. Soon I have done enough. I take the jug back, carefully and proudly, to Carol like a kitten who has caught a rat, to find I was only supposed to use the jug to measure it. Carol didn't need to see more of my urine, she trusted me to tell her the amount. Whoops.

Carol is kind though. She knows I'm tired. It is only a week later that I realise the humiliating truth – I spent ages wandering around a large hospital with a jug of my own warm piss. I should have kept it for visitors, like Samuel Pepys.

She scans my bladder with a probe on my belly to see if anything has been retained and gives us some instructions about starting my pelvic floor exercises again and when we need to come back, which my mum writes down because they've gone from my mind in an instant. Then she asks if I would mind if the student nurse who was at my appointment earlier this morning comes back in to see.

I am past caring how many people look at my shame, prod it and touch it, but I'm perturbed. I'm feeling fairly chatty now and, I notice, not sitting in such a forced and weird position. Which test have I failed now that the nurse may need to look at? My mum squeezes my hand.

'Look,' says Carol as they walk back in.

'Yes,' replies the nurse.

'A different woman,' says Carol gently.

'I wouldn't recognise her,' concurs the student.

They are right. Free of the bag, sore and in need of rest, haggard from a week of nonsense, and yet I'm smiling again. The swelling goes down. The pain eases. I am changed.

What emerges, again, is not Venus radiant in her shell, nor a phoenix smouldering out of ash into life. Hell, this time it's not even something fully fixed and ready for a new baby, but it is something good-ish, and new-ish for me. And that's important.

The thing is, an operation is a mindfuck, but a lot of patient information skips over the reality, perhaps because it might scare people off electing for a surgery that could be a massive help. Don't be scared. If an op is the right thing for you, and you understand and are happy with the benefits *and* the risks, then think about it. Just don't expect to spring out of bed the next morning.

If it isn't the right thing for you, there will be other options, so try to remember that action of any kind – turning up, doing your exercises, talking to experts, researching your condition, getting second opinions – these are important and valid. Not least as they prove to yourself that you are worth the fight.

Part Four

THE FINAL
TABOOS

Chapter 17

Potty training

I call 2013–14 the lost years. My diaries and hospital letters spill the worst secrets as I try to stay sane and chipper. This period starts slowly as we 'watch and wait' to see how and if my operation has actually worked. This is as boring as it is infuriating, not least as the answer is 'quite a bit' rather than 'YES COMPLETELY'. I haven't got my perfect happy ending, one where my boys, Carol, my husband and I pogo off together into the sunset like a dry-knickered *Famous Five*. Instead of a 'new normal', a 'clean slate', I end up with a continence relapse that starts with an over-productive fart.

Worse, before I can even bring myself to start tackling a decline in one sort of continence running hand in hand with some improvement in the other, I am confronted by something new. How do I successfully potty train a child when I cannot lead by example? How do I encourage him not to make a mess, without explicitly humiliating him? The answer is badly.

The first time round, we read up on it. We even set up a special 'potty rug' so my son knew where to go. It wasn't massively successful. We trained him like a cat, so if the potty was being bleached elsewhere, he would just happily do his business in the corner of the room, agog if we suggested that wasn't the agreement.

The second time we knew better, and, due to that and all the medical faffing, we waited until he could talk. I may now be an advocate for increasing the conversation around continence but this was my worst idea ever.

August/September 2013, toy- and tantrum-strewn landscape that was once a hopeful love nest

He's always seen me coming, and pounced on any sign of intellectual weakness, but potty training is turning out to be my second child's *tour de force*. It's a race to the bottom from the start. Even the new exciting big boy pants I purchase are interpreted as a challenge – which of his favourite TV characters would *I* prefer he defile? (Poor, poor Fireman Sam.)

He is an aggressive, literal pint-sized philosopher, cutting to shreds the euphemisms and inaccuracies in the way we talk about toilets. One day, after breakfast he looks up, impervious.

'We don't wee on the kitchen chair,' I say, gamely, with only a hint of annoyance as I wipe up the watery mess and discover last week's Weetabix welded to the seat.

'I just did,' he corrects, with disdain.

'You can't go around just pooing on the floor!' I try later, trying to remain upbeat as I skirt around him, cleaning up shit in between loading the washing machine.

'Yes I can,' he says, as his little mound seeps between the floor-boards. 'LOOK!'

'Are you doing a poo or a trump?' I shriek desperately at bedtime, running towards him as he crouches down ominously by his bed.

'YES,' he shouts, as if he'll never meet a bigger moron. 'YES, I AM DOING A POO OR A TRUMP.'

At the time, I have no idea how it will end. I stay hopeful about pants before school, but this thought reminds me once again of how easily we take the good luck of continence for granted, those of us blessed with it from an early age. But I would like to avoid any more crap around the house – and I have a nagging doubt this would be over far quicker if I told him he was disgusting and unloveable when he dirtied the carpet.

Potty training involves introducing cherubic toddlers to the idea that the sun does not shine out of their perfect bottoms. For many, this is a sudden *volte-face*. They must learn that certain fluids and behaviours are not acceptable in public, even if Mummy and Daddy know they are natural and normal. The same mummy and daddy who have in fact spent the child's entire life so far stuffing their noses in their nappies in restaurants to take a massive sniff.

I don't remember the first time I learned about control, but my mother says I was potty trained at around two-and-a-half so it was probably late 1979.

'It was the snowman knickers that did it, so it must have been winter!' she adds.

In the early twentieth century, mothers were encouraged to teach babies good and clean habits, holding even tiny ones over a chamber pot to encourage weeing in the right place. This messy method, given how much babies and toddlers wriggle, assumed women would be working themselves to death on boiling laundry 24/7 anyway. Perhaps the laundry is why, though, being un-messy was such an urgent life goal.

US guru Doctor Benjamin Spock, credited with changing many child-rearing ideas, advocated learning without such force. He was clear that parents shouldn't bang on about how disgusting or awful toilet accidents are in case the child absorbed those ideas as criticisms of themselves. My mum took her parenting advice from paediatrician Hugh Jolly, whose books suggested letting your child train himself and remaining sceptical when listening to didactic potty-training methods. I too have found almost all advice about potty training to be pissing in the wind. Endless readings of *I Want My Potty* were as useful as dreamcatchers for my poor sleepers, or those snoring lion clocks that growl white noise and end up as a £30 doorstop.

My mother doesn't remember any particularly traumatic piddling from me, though she does say I always used to wet the bed when we stayed at other people's houses, and this early incontinence I do remember. Feeling the warmth and the release and then the shivery truth when you wee in your sleep is a common problem. Regular wetting affects boys slightly more than girls, and in rare cases continues into adulthood. It can happen to old and young people under certain circumstances, such as if they are poorly or drunk. Most of us have probably been there. It's the stuff of rockstar autobiographies. If you are famous enough, you can style anything out. I don't remember it being okay for me. I can still feel the itch, and recall peeling off my polyester nightie like a price sticker, cold and limp. And the simple horror of the 'Oh God, not again' feeling that rippled over my gut, like the goosebumps on my skin.

I also remember picking my moment for confession. Because it felt like a confession in the light of a brand-new day. It wasn't fair to tell Mummy and Daddy straight away, when they first woke up. I used to wait until after we'd all had a nice morning cuddle in their bed and snuggling into their sheets had warmed me up.

Writing about bedwetting reminds me of something worse – the nightmare of wetting the bed, climbing in with your folks and then all falling back to sleep. Sometimes you only remember to tell at your next bedtime, when you catch a whiff of wee as you slip back onto the damp patch.

Regular bedwetting is a relatively common form of incontinence. Studies quoted by NICE and the NHS show just over one in five children wets the bed at four and a half. And just under one in 12 still do at nine and a half.

The trouble for me is that I remember the waterproof sheet, but not the milestone of not needing it. I wish one of us had written it down, then I could have calculated how many perfectly decent continent years I had before my pelvic flaws(!) came to light.

Being toilet trained is so fundamental to our growing up that when it goes – and you know you really might leave the worst kind of damp patch on the bed, and you are too old to be *that* drunk student with a spreading stain on your trousers and too young to be in a care home – what then? When you have an operation that was supposed to fix it, how do you cope or understand it when that doesn't work in the way that you'd hoped? If I'd saved the sticker chart, I could have consoled myself that I mastered it once.

Maybe I could have removed the stress, rather than my sense of self, or felt inspired to get better. Instead, my leaking made me mournful. But something was happening as that year tumbled into the next that was about to take me to the heart of the taboo. I was about to hit rock bottom. Emphasis on the second word.

Chapter 18

Poo

There's a lot to say about poo, both from a parenting perspective and if we're looking critically at incontinence and taboo. Poo incontinence is terrifying – as bodily mishaps go, the fear of wetting yourself is probably only eclipsed by the dread of publicly following through on a fart. But even for those of us who can't make jokes about sweetcorn, parenting forces us into a scatological mindset. The truest sign of being a new parent, after all, is looking in the mirror and thinking: 'God, what's that shit on my face?' only to realise: 'Oh GOD. It's shit. On my face!'

One of the few things that kept me from actually teetering into the abyss for the first few incontinent years was being able to answer the worst questions, the ones about my bowels, with a definite NO. I wouldn't be alone. Poo is, primally, connected with our sensation and experience of disgust. Faeces is a 'Core Disgust Elicitor', and child psychologists have diligently documented the exact developmental stage where children will recoil from a chocolate shaped like a turd, rather than wolfing it down. The moment where the horror of the sticky stuff finally kicks in. Disgust is worse than mere distaste too – it has a moral dimension, it is a reaction to something wholly bad.

I am definitely disgusted and disgruntled when I first crap myself. One brown accident and like Keyser Söze, like a breath in the wind, like it never really existed at all, my last sliver of dignity was gone.

'All this, ALL THIS, and the op didn't even fucking work completely,' I think, smarting from such an unfair hand. I doubt I would have taken it with much grace if it had happened to me at any point in life, in any case, but it was hard not to descend to the pits, although I know I tried various techniques to cope. I regularly bought treats on the way back from hospital or spent the whole tube home retelling the story in my head until it disappeared or took shape as a shocking but hilarious anecdote.

I barely spoke about it though. And I didn't write about it because the whole experience would have sounded like a fanciful and messy dream. Which is odd, because it started on a very ordinary, boring Saturday, when I didn't even think I needed the toilet.

Summer 2013, rebuilding a normal life in a messy kitchen

I'm drinking tea with my husband as the children nap. We're still potty training so there's toilet trappings everywhere but we're ignoring the mess and doing a quiz in the paper. We're sitting at the large oak table we bought when we were young lovers. It's the one piece of furniture left from our twenties that's compatible with family life, and which we haven't gone off in the meantime. It has matching oak chairs, with fabric seats. At that table we are proper grown-ups.

I reach for a Hobnob, and then it happens. I suddenly shit myself. I start, but I can't stop. It seeps through my clothes and onto the chair. I thought it was a gurgle or some wind I could hang onto, but I couldn't. It wasn't. I'm horrified. I'm like my son when he stands defiant near a pair of soiled pants, all of us staring at his moussey offerings. I wonder if I can get upstairs without my husband noticing, but I am rooted to the spot. I hear a cracking sound – rwack – but it's not the chair, it's a wire springing loose in my mind. I have visions of oozing and mess but it doesn't matter, because I'm frozen.

'Babe,' my husband asks, 'why are you crying?'

I try to explain, but I can't admit it. Though I'm also wondering: *who am I trying to fool?*

I think back. In the hell of surgery recovery I wasn't brave enough to assess my knicker mess. Since then it's been creeping in. Denial. I've just been chucking most of it away without looking to check what is in it: pads, crinkly disposable knickers, sometimes real knickers. The more I bin, I realise, the less I look. I stopped analysing what's been leaking from where in that last infection. Even though I did have nagging doubts about skid marks.

I know why I couldn't confront it – *because I am to blame.* I have a guilty secret: I've not been doing my exercises properly. I've done them, yes, but not religiously every day. I knew pelvic floors were a life-long commitment for someone like me. Christ knows, Lizzie drummed it into me, kindly. But somehow, after the op, as I started leaking again, little by little, I started to resent the idea that they were mine to do 'for the rest of my life'.

'I've been a wanker and I've let my bottom collapse,' I want to howl, realising I've been in a permanent snark with the Waz Wizard and co, who've left the hard boring work to me. That's self-pity for you.

I can't remember how we cleared the poo up. I think I insisted on doing it myself. I can remember thinking, 'Oh God, Brett, properly broken now,' as I stand at the sink, rubbing soap so far under my fingernails they bend back into creased half-moons in the steam. I try and try to scrub and scald the dirt away. And then, still numb, march into the lounge and order some tasteful plastic dining chairs online. You know, *just in case.*

I could start the exercises again (and I did) but rebuilding faith in the future was harder. I didn't really *expect* the operation to be a cure-all, but a part of me felt I deserved it to be, that I was owed an all-mended 'ta-dah' moment. I wonder if that was what

I was hoping for (or expecting?) when I started my incontinence blog, which now stood fallow too. A happy nappy ending? How complacent I was. How naive! I can admit it now.

I was lucky though, because institutions took over. Because my history meant I had a hospital number and people who saw me fast. People who listened, and believed me, and sent me on a grand tour of imaging departments where every aspect of my bottom was put under the microscope.

LUCKY.

Late summer 2013, arriving for a bum balloon test in my lunchbreak

I enter the office of a bowel specialist. For her test, she will insert a balloon into my bottom. This makes me feel like a circus act, an inverted novelty machine. I have to tell her when I can feel pressure.

As it inflates, I want to give her the right answer, but I don't know what she's looking for. A tickle, a touch, some key sensation? Eventually, I feel a bit like something's pressing me.

'Now!' I say.

'Really?' she asks, like I'm insane. I correct myself and try to try harder. I shout 'NOW' again, after extra inflation. She looks quizzical but notes it down. I don't want to know my score. I won't understand it and I suspect I will feel bad either way – the result will either be normal so I'll look like I'm faking, or it won't and I will have to accept I'm broken. I blubber.

'You aren't helpless,' she says, as I wipe snot on my sleeve. 'And it won't always feel this bad. We'll get to the bottom of this.'

That week, I cut my long brown hair off. I say to Cat, 'After the arse balloon, I had to do *something* that felt proactive, and radical, and not about continence.'

It's a start.

Autumn 2013, the return to Urogynaecology

Both the initial balloon test results and my new bob look great, I'm told, and there's no evidence or suggestion that the op caused the issue. I'm back with Carol and co, and though we all know it is probably a result of my now catastrophically demotivated and exhausted pelvic floor, they vow to investigate (and eliminate) anything else nasty that might be going on. They are here for me.

Carol even has products that might help control the issue in the interim, including, wait for it: bum tampons (aka anal plugs).

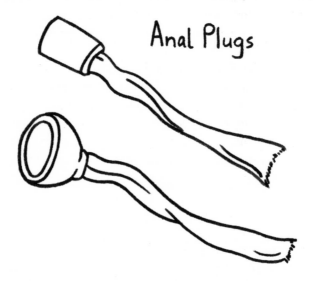

Anal Plugs

Made out of a soft foam with a gauzy string to pull it out, the Peristeen anal plug is marketed as a 'simple, safe and discreet aid for faecal incontinence … [that] prevents the uncontrolled loss of solid stool … can easily fit into your pocket or handbag … [and] cannot be seen by others as it is worn inside the body'. Not only does it stop poo leaking out, the blurb adds, 'unpleasant odours are also avoided'. Tidy.

You insert them like a suppository, which is easy as they are compressed to the size of a hazelnut and coated with a water-soluble film. You lube it up and pop it in, then the film dissolves in the warmth of your bottom and the plug expands to fit snugly in your rectal cavity. Other brands are available.

'It's like a cork,' I say, in shock and amazement. 'A cork for my bum!'

Carol smiles and doles out a fistful of samples and some sachets of lube. She warns me about the websites where I can order them; she can see maybe that it will be too much for me to scroll past the pouches, compact catheters and silicon sheaths just now.

I want to ask if they ever fall out – I don't want *that* in my pants if I laugh too hard – but it feels like nit-picking so I shove the samples in my handbag and say thank you. I won't use them unless it gets really bad.

When I see the Waz Wizard he gives me a tissue, which makes me cry more as it feels like I've levelled up to a new part of the grimness game. He waits for me to stop juddering, and tells me he's sending me to see another nurse practitioner who works in a related department.

Janice is my magic ass nurse. She's cut from the same cloth as Carol, but with more diagrams of shit on the walls of her office. She pushes through with no truck for denial, desperation or discomfiture – her mission is to improve our pooing habits and she will not succumb to any ickiness.

She re-introduces me to the Bristol Stool Form Scale that Jenny showed me right at the start (*see also* page 84), so I can point out my cracked sausages and soft blobs again, and acts like we're exchanging shopping tips when we talk straining (very bad for the pelvic floor), evacuation speed (I know!), diet, farts and bottom strength. I think it's especially kind of her, given I have changed status now – I am panicking and I have a problem, but I am by no means 'off the scale' in here; I'm one of her easier patients.

I'm so basic she has to teach me how to poo. She shows me how to mimic squatting, using a stool or a rolled-up bath towel under my feet to lift them up so my hips are not at a 90-degree angle and I am no longer just sitting on the pan. This helps straighten out the kink where the colon and rectum join and allows the motion to pass more easily. She suggests leaning forwards too, elbows on knees, so I am in a squatting pose but also sitting on the loo. I do not want to know what I look like, though I think I'm a faintly ridiculous homage to Eddie The Eagle – another lovable loser about to take flight. A semi-nude ski-jumper on the edge of glory, or oblivion. Another physio suggests making a noise as I poo might help reduce straining, but I'm not sure if I can sing along just yet.

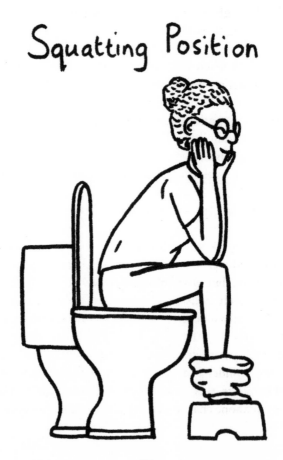

Squatting Position

I have to go on a bland diet, avoiding high fibre, nuts, alcohol and sweeteners like sorbitol. It's boring and a bit like nursery food, white bread and no flavour, but it calms things down.

Only one bad thing happens at Janice's bum clinic and it doesn't happen in her room. On my third visit, I walk into the waiting area and see someone I know. It's a friend's sister.

I freeze. Do I say hello? What's the etiquette for the degree of intimacy revealed by our shared clinic number? Which bit of life school covered that? Did I miss it?

I go for a gentle nod, and duck down to look at a magazine. I hide behind the glossy pages and run through the options again and again, trying to work out what's best.

Of all my experiences with Janice, this is the most perturbing – even more than when she made me act out a poo and told me I'd been doing it wrong my whole life. I still feel incredibly sad when I think of that day. How I wish I'd been brave enough to wave, start a conversation, show solidarity. How I wish I'd been better. And how hard I hope that the other patient knew I wasn't being dismissive, or thinking she was disgusting or wanting to perpetuate the stigma. How I hope she realised that I just didn't know how to say anything at all, that I couldn't find the right words then, because for me at that point, there weren't any.

Janice wrong-foots me that day too, by bringing up constipation. Something that affects my bladder, pushing my prolapse down, but that I hadn't linked to my leaking poo. Counterintuitively, constipation can cause leaks when runny poo explodes around a blocked one. She says my ski-jumper position will help.

I close my eyes as she says this, as if it will hide my burning cheeks, and wonder how the hell I will answer her questions about things like this at our next appointment, a scheduled weekday telephone chat, which I'll have to do sitting in my open-plan office.

Winter 2013, GP office, the worst prescription ever

'It's a racket,' shrieks my GP, incredulous, as she reads the price of the bum tampons – £2 a unit – for the NHS while filling in my prescription.

I try comradery and a knowing joke.

'It's almost as if they're so shameful, it's easy to rack the price up as no one will complain,' I laugh. But I think I'm letting the side down, and she can probably see it in my face.

'I don't resent it for people like you, who need them,' she adds (to reassure?). I want to sulk about the 'people like you' comment but I'm distracted by her attitude. My GP's not embarrassed, she's positively enthusiastic about anal plugs. Maybe because she's a body mechanic at heart, she's unabashedly intrigued about how they work and what they look like.

I don't often get to help doctors do anything, so I offer her my last sample, which is still hiding in my handbag in its slippy green wrapper.

She's like a child at Christmas.

She plays with it like Rik Mayall in *The Young Ones* with his tampon mouse, and then turns back to her PC. She pauses.

'Oh dear,' she says. 'The computer needs to know your size.'

'SMALL,' I shout, before I can stop myself. *Dear God, please make me a small.*

The idea of large ones is just too much. Too much. And then I burst. Ugly crying. My face is a mess. I'm no hot tramp – I'm a broken gargoyle. I almost make a neighing sound as the ancient printer churns out my prescription.

'I think it is making me really depressed again,' I say, to lighten the mood and distract from the wailing. 'I don't think I can carry on. I think I'm broken now.'

'I'm not surprised,' she replies, and offers to sign me off work until I can at least start the tests and work out how to cope. I'm not sure I dare take time off, but I can see she might be right. The truth is I am sick and I need help. All because of a bit of poo.

I feel like a loser, but I am having panic attacks about crapping myself. Crying myself to sleep. Not able to bear looking at my knickers when I do leak. And hyperventilating whenever I get a hospital letter that details another invasive test.

'Does everyone get so upset about it?' I ask. Maybe there's a flaw in my thinking we can mend, something we can fix.

'To be honest,' she says, 'people hardly ever talk about it. They can't. In 20 years, you are one of the only patients I've had who has spoken about the emotional side of it at all, Luce.'

Every doctor I meet accepts the obviousness of a nervous break-down with faecal laxity. Most people do, if they think about it.

My colleague Ally sees me burst into tears trying to book an appointment online that has 'colon' in the title. She hugs me and says, 'That's. Just. Horrible.'

It might not be Shakespeare but it's a relief to hear someone else agree. And that she touched me without recoiling. Even my boss, who has seen my deterioration but not known why, is gracious when I have an accident on the way home from work and decide to take my GP up on some recovery time.

I tearfully speak to HR and then email my line manager saying I can't carry on, that I now have terrible incontinence problems and I don't know how to sort them out. I say it affects everyday tasks from getting dressed, to travelling, to long meetings and apologise for the subject matter being disgusting. I get an email back the next morning. It's kind and helpful and direct. He says he's pleased I told him, and acknowledges it can't have been easy to write to him at all. And his focus is on rebuilding – he says we can work out what can be done to make my work life easier and enable me to cope and recover. I keep his reply for a long time. Not because he's kind (although he is), or because it makes me feel relieved, but because it represents something about finally admitting it all and having a straightforward dialogue about what was happening to me with someone non-medical. It showed me that even with the cat out of the bag there *were* people who would help, even if my condition was messy and hard to talk about. I'm not sure how to describe the milestone, though. Courage, maybe? The start of telling my truth?

That was all just treading water before the real trials began. Soon it was time for my tests to truly take over – more explorations to find out whether anything sinister underlies my leaking. I can only detail them very quickly so we can all hear them once and then forget about it. But at least then you'll know about the sort of things that can happen, and how to avoid the worst bits, if you ever need to. Heaven knows, I'd have liked to have known what I was in for.

Winter 2013, colonoscopy, gastro department full of bottom doctors in scrubs

Colonoscopies are common. And they are fine. Mine didn't hurt and the prep was worse than the poking. It was also the easiest to talk about as a lot of people have had them. My friend Scott gave some good advice, along with gleeful descriptions of his own experience of the test when he was urged to try and fart in front of some nurses.

'You'd do anything for your kids, so you must do anything to take care of yourself so you can be there for them. Even this, Luce,' he says, before offering a play-by-play of the two-day prep, the weirdly restrictive bland diet, the mounting tension as you drink pints of liquid laxative, and the astonishing sensation of shitting everything you've ever eaten (or thought about eating) until nothing but clear water is pouring out.

The wait for the anal avalanche is quite something, agrees another friend online. But the more extensive, the better. If you are at all competitive, you can take pride in having shiny clean lip-pink caverns showing up on the monitor as the doctor feeds a camera up and looks at you inside as you lie back, calmed down and drugged up.

Colonoscopies are also fine because you have to take someone with you. Not to watch the imaging of your inners, but because you have been sedated so can't drive.

Next up was a scan of the muscles around my anus. It was also totally fine. The staff were sweet and the scan – not unlike an early pregnancy ultrasound – only took minutes, using a well-lubricated and narrow wand-like probe. I can honestly say, if you need one, have one.

But if possible, maybe don't go on your own. You can't always suspend your dignity and expect to bounce back seconds later.

Winter 2013, after the anal scan, mysterious imaging suite, big familiar hospital

I'm not sure quite when I lurched through a tear in the fabric of time. One second, I was wiping some lube from my bum crack and saying thank you (*ALWAYS SAY THANK YOU, LUCE – NOBODY ASKED TO LOOK AT YOUR BOTTOM*) and the next, I was kneeling in one of the patient toilets, rocking.

I'd had a baby here, physiotherapy, the op; it was so familiar, but I was lost. Utterly. The toilet looked like all the others, except this time I was hunched in a ball. Keening. It lasted so long that when I left, I wondered if I'd been locked in.

I spent a quarter of an hour wandering around. I was in a different imaging department, a different wing, a different set of lifts and stairs. It was the middle of the night now. And dark hospitals can be so freaky and disorientating in their sameness. Especially when you can only think that someone has just put one of those condom-covered probes up your bottom and you thanked them for it. I could hardly breathe as I ran across a glass bridge, when, thank God, I saw the front doors.

The next thing I knew, that I really knew must be true, was the bright sunshine. I was sitting on a metal bench in one of the large

London squares. Sobbing. Again. In public. Again. And it wasn't the middle of the night. It wasn't even evening. It was still the afternoon. How could I have got so confused? I was baffled by where and when I was.

'Do you think your PTSD might be back?' asked my friend, a doctor.

Certainly, there were similarities with my previous experiences and diagnosis. Again, I'd hurtled back in time. I was the little one shitting their pants in the reading corner. Knowing deep down, even at four years old, that the mob would remember my name, my shame, as long as I would.

I knew, objectively, I was a grown-up with an embarrassing health complaint, but I'd spend hours panicking about whether my skin was stained, or if that was just ageing, terrified I'd leave a trace and the doctors would think I just couldn't wipe my bum.

Sometimes before appointments I even scrubbed my bottom with household cleaners. How's that for self-harm, wiping with Ecover just to try and get it clean? But that was the fear. That I would be an appalling display.

And worse, I wasn't just ashamed *of me*. I was horrified *for them*.

'Poor, poor fuckers,' I used to think. 'How do they get up in the morning?'

How awful for them, watching me roll over to stare at the wall as they parted my cheeks to insert something – a finger? A balloon? A hamster? I never did get a Freddie Starr joke in there.

I know a psychoanalyst who was a nurse in her first career. She is shocked when I 'fess up to all this worry.

She tells me nurses, doctors, imaging specialists, physiotherapists often go into those professions *because* they have an interest in the tactile, the bodily. They like taste, smell, sensation, touch. Bodies do not revolt them – farts, noises, moving genitals, these

are clues that give them information. My body horror wasn't
something they shared.

My doctor friend concurred: 'We like touching and looking at
broken bodies – because it makes us feel dead clever when we can
fix them.'

I just about manage to park my fear and revulsion, until the
letter arrives.

Spring 2014, the MRI money shot

The hospital has written, inviting me to an MRI proctogram. I
read the phrase 'MRI proctogram', imagine I have made it up,
and read it again. Yup. It is a thing.

I know MRIs are a bit awful, I've had one before. Survivable,
but like the physical embodiment of a migraine in an enclosed
space. And I know about proctologists because of all the jokes
in American movies about doctors who stick their finger up
your bottom.

I stand stock-still in the hall. Like I'm in a movie myself, staring at the paper in front of me. It's as if a committee has devised
the worst, most humiliating and horrible test to inflict on my
beleaguered psyche.

I glance at it in case any details jump out, details that will not
confirm my fear that I might actually have to go to the toilet in the
middle of a magnetic machine.

My low-level medical Latin was on the money though. This is
what they want me to do. I go to the patient info sheet; maybe I'll
find something reassuring there. I find something worse. Idiocy.
Some people (*some people!*), it says, find the test embarrassing and
upsetting, but it isn't those things.

I want to scream.

They are going to film me pooing. I already know from reading
the description that it will be embarrassing *and* upsetting, for me
at least and no doubt pretty messy too. What they mean, I think

(hope?), is that it isn't shameful, and patients shouldn't think they will disgust anyone working there. I think they should also add reassurance that even if you cry your hardest you won't short circuit the machine, to ward off my panic that I'll blow myself up before I even drop my load.

It isn't even at my regular hospital, so I won't know any of the staff – I can't decide if this is a blessing or a curse.

I post on an online forum and let my husband read the letter, goggle-eyed. I want to sound out my fears but it is so surreal, it sounds magical. I even consider talking to my toilet-humour obsessed children about it; they'll probably relish the chance to hear about something that rude, I think. But in the end I don't dare, because of SHAME. And because I'm too frightened they might see my chance to shit on a table in public as the final proof that grown-ups are monstrous hypocrites who save all the cool stuff for themselves.

The day starts well, with a nice big enema. The nurse is perfunctory, like the setting. There are no cubicles so once she has pumped my bottom full of a special liquid (via a nozzle attached to a pouch that looks a lot like a hot water bottle) I have to wait for it to 'take hold' in the public waiting room and then when it does, and I get the sharp pain that means I need to run to a loo, I have to hotfoot it to the public conveniences. The liquid is specifically designed to loosen things up so I will fully evacuate my bowels. Knowing this is imminent while sitting in the waiting room is not relaxing. I almost collapse into hysterics when, after a particularly close shave, I finally get it all out and the nurse checks me and declares me 'clean'.

I'm sent into the MRI room to change into a gown, and then another nurse and a man whose job title I don't know ask me to lie down so they can fill me with a special jelly, which will show up on their screens. It's okay, they say, they have locked the door.

The man is dishy, and I have to look away from his face when he talks. Then he starts to squeeze glow-in-the-dark gloop up my passage. I'm beyond small talk. The jelly insertion is discombob-ulating, and cold.

I hear a sigh. The professionals stop to talk, and yes, they agree, just one bag of jelly isn't enough. I have a bigger than average bum hole.

'OH GOD,' I think, as my soul evaporates. 'I AM full of shit after all.' *Still got it.*

They explained what is about to happen: I'll be lying in the machine, but to ensure they can see the motions *accurately*, I will need to be sort of tied to a special booster seat with a hole in it. Strapped in tightly so I can't move. Like an astronaut with no knickers.

I stare at them.

I can't just go willy-nilly, they say, I have to wait for their signal. But don't worry, they will tell me when to get started, when the machine has warmed up and moved me into place.

They give me a button to press if I want to stop the test at any time. I press the button. The technician laughs. We all do.

'It's for when you're in there,' he says.

'I know,' I think, but I want to get the jelly out of my bum, STAT. So I saddle up and listen to jazz over the headphones. The dishy technician talks me through the whole thing. This is comforting until I start my poo and have to tell him to stop being so encouraging. I can't have a running commentary as the gloop moulds into a pseudo-shit and edges onto the padded sheet. It's too grim.

And then it's over. They tell me that the recording is great. Very clear. I pretend to be thrilled at their expert work, though I'll be honest, it doesn't feel great and I fear it being used in train-ing as an example scan.

The nurse comes in with a cardboard bowl and some paper towels and I have to wipe myself down and then dash to the disabled loo again to get dressed. The technician is very nice, but I fear that the department has taken destigmatising one level too far. To something closer to indifference. It's as if they've forgotten how any of this might actually feel.

Because surely everyone knows the fear factor of involuntary bowel evacuation?

When I was in my early twenties, Manchester United manager Alex Ferguson used the risk of diarrhoea to get off a speeding charge. His lawyer was widely quoted at the time as saying his client had to speed on the M602 because the alternative was 'unthinkable'. The bench agreed. Public poo is *unthinkable*.

We are so weird about illness and bodies anyway, but especially bottoms. We're so hung up about it that people die because they can't talk about it – or feel ashamed of themselves when they are sick or dying, and deserve to be bathed in love and compassion.

When she was dying, actress Lynda Bellingham said her bowel cancer wasn't one of the 'sexy cancers', not one people spoke about. She said that's what motivated her to speak about it during her last weeks and months, to encourage people to look out for their bowels and not let the stigma stop them getting screenings or talking to doctors. It made me weep, partly because I thought I knew her in the marrow of my being, from the Oxo adverts where she was a beleaguered mum and comforter to an entire nation through the '80s and '90s, but also because it is so true.

We treat bottoms with such fear and contempt, despite the brilliantly brutal statistic that around *one in 10 of us will suffer from involuntary poo leaking at some point in our lives*!

In a 2016 study Dr Emily Rubin in Pennsylvania showed that over two-thirds (68.9 per cent) of seriously ill patients considered bowel and bladder incontinence to be grimmer (or the same) as meeting the Grim Reaper himself. Jeez, Louise, what a fucking mess we are in!

Though it is published well after I hit the eye of the storm, the research is fascinating because it is so shocking. First, it demonstrates in the starkest, and somehow saddest, terms that the secret fear that many incontinent people share – that everyone else is filled with pity, disgust and dread at the thought of being anything like us – is based in fact. Many people would rather die than share our fate. Brilliant.

Secondly, it justifies the need for more investment, and commitment, to challenge our instincts to hide this stuff away. We are an ageing global population now, dying later, and with older pelvic floors and sphincters than previous civilisations could ever have imagined. We're surviving childbirth injury and we've learned enough about numbers to work out one in 10 of us will leak poo. So we need to get a grip and find a way to move on from this silly, silly fucking fear.

But thirdly, as the study is based on a hypothetical idea rather than reality, it can't be telling the whole story, can it?

When the poo tests are done and dusted, nothing more terrible has been found, and everyone agrees that the best course of action for now is strengthening my pelvic floor, using aids when needed, and carrying on carrying on, I look further.

There must be another set of stories out there, some good, some bad, some ugly. Stories of how people actually did cope, and did not die of shame, when they became incontinent. The study highlights colossal negative impressions of the impact on patients' quality of life and mental health. But it didn't ask people who actually live with dual incontinence whether they would rather be dead. It wasn't focused only on people who knew what it was like. Anyone can guess, based on fear and taboo, what double incontinence might mean; that doesn't really tell us much about how it is to be doubly incontinent. For some patients – those for whom incontinence has always been a part of their life, or those for whom a catastrophic event or illness, such as spinal damage or brain damage, has removed any chance of regaining control – there is, potentially, a quite different story.

In those circumstances, incontinence often just has to be considered for what it is: an ultimately mechanical problem, albeit one that can cause distress; a distress which, thanks to the stigma, cannot always be soothed.

This thought inspires me to seek out the good news stories, the stigma-smashers, the innovators. From new products like low 'rustle', leak-proof clothes to artists and photographers making ostomies look beautiful; from awareness weeks, charities and forums to ordinary, inspirational incontinent people picking their self-esteem up, dusting it down and ploughing on with pads or rubber trousers, or bags and specialist underwear.

Surely, I too can learn to find some form of acceptance of my position.

Summer 2014, a small boy's bedroom, evening

The night is perfect. We've read *The Very Angry Ladybird* and played at being kings. His Spider-Man pyjamas are a second skin, which make me love him more. I know he needs to go to sleep but I relish these evening chats when I'm just back from work and I am compelled to make him laugh, not calm him down. My boy.

Desperate for his laughter, I play our favourite game. I sit on the bed, poised to tickle and declare war, shouting: 'Who's the boss?'

'I am,' he replies, thrilled at the indiscretion.

'The cheek of it! Who's the boss?' I demand.

'I am.'

'You ratbag!' I say, tickling deep. 'Who's the boss?'

'I AM!'

He's squealing and letting out airy yelps. A pipe organ. A steam train's whistle. Swallowing his laughs so hard he'll get indigestion. 'Stop, Mummy. STOP.'

I let us breathe but have to ask, 'Do you remember who the boss is now?'

'Yes.'

'WHO THEN?'

'Grandma.'

He screams at my outrage. We roll off the bed and around the carpet. A mock battle, arms, legs, curls fly around amongst the giggles.

'Sometimes I think you are just a beast,' I say. 'You know Mummy is the all-knowing, all-loving God of the universe.'

'How much do you love me?' he asks, always the pint-sized philosopher, my toddler sage. 'To the moon and back?'

'More than that,' I retort. 'More than that. To the bottom of the sea where Captain Barnacles explores and up into the sky until there's nothing but stars. To the moon and back? The moon and back? Pah! I love you back to the beginning of time.'

'Do you love everything about me?'

'Everything.'

'My stinky feet?' he shouts, offering them up.

'Yes!' I shout back and dive in for a lick.

'My shoulder pit?'

'Yes.'

He's enjoying this.

'My knees?'

'Of course your knees!' I shriek.

And then, not skipping a beat: 'Even the poo in my bum, Mummy?'

He's got me. Again. I'm the patsy. His eyes are wide. Cracked coal. Dark crystals.

'Even the poo in your bum,' I admit.

Because it's the truth. Perhaps that's what love means after all.

Chapter 19

Stigma

Though we get the poo relatively under control, those lost years start to stretch out, contributing to a sense that I'd been further robbed of my thirties. The cumulative mess doesn't help my state of mind. And then I have a breakthrough, on my birthday in June 2014, when I crack my right femur stumbling off a curb. Somehow this is the impetus I need – along with the fear I'll be stuck leaking forever – to force me to tackle the stigma up close. Not least as I can start by testing the hypothesis that embarrassing health issues should be, as everyone keeps saying to me, 'just like a broken leg'.

The fractured foot hurts and the boot I have to wear is slippy on floorboards and makes accidents more likely, adding pressure to my stitched-up bladder neck and leaving me in full-time pads again. I briefly experience functional incontinence – like the elderly people who don't quite make it as they rush for the loo. I know I need it; I just can't get there fast enough with one leg clad in plastic and Velcro.

But mainly it proves what I'd always expected. Broken legs are nothing like a broken bladder or a broken mind. With my leg, sympathy is easy and direct. People offer seats and practical things – they don't get so tied up in their own feelings that they can't be helpful. Nobody blushes. They don't share intimate details of their own lives or their mothers', or think twice about whether I am a good mum. Nobody comments on my health choices or circumstances, or says they don't believe in X-rays and bandages with the same vigour they tell me they don't believe in therapy or antidepressants. And no one thinks I am a posh mum having a strop or I should just do more Pilates and hide that I'm bummed out. It's easier to tell my male colleagues too.

Annoyingly though, the problem with this kind of intro-spection is that it makes it too easy to become angry with those around you, bitter even, that nobody quite knows what to say but you still have to deal with it all. It makes it too easy to forget that they are just as sullied as you are by the stigma surrounding continence and mental health.

I want to find my people, others who understand living with the stigma and all it steals, to hear other voices tell me their stories that sound like mine.

It first happens with Jeanette Winterson. Reading her memoir *Why Be Happy When You Could Be Normal?* (incredible question!) is the first time I feel it. The sharp gut relief of recognition as I'm holding a paperback engrossed in a story.

She hits a crisis point searching for her birth mother, and sinks to the floor in her own kitchen and wets herself (as a middle-aged woman). Winterson has written about bodies before. In *Oranges Are Not The Only Fruit*, and all her early work with its knickers and sex and honesty, and *Written On The Body*, which seems to talk direct to the shy patient in me.

I wish.

And she's reluctant to tell about her accident. The watery mess that pulls together all the ideas of childhood, transitions, independence and domestic space that her story throws up. She really sounds ashamed. I want to touch her fingertips and connect.

Her story is so raw it reminds me of another autobiographi-cal work I read years ago: Frank Skinner's eponymous memoir, where he describes his alcoholism. Skinner presents his drunken bedwetting as key to his rock-bottom, complete with emphatic bouts of denial about waking with a dry mouth and a wet bed.

It's like they know the truth, as I am also discovering it – their shame is frozen in time, waiting for me to find it. They know you can pretty much always clear up piss with a glug of Dettol, but the stigma leaves its mark for far longer. I can't ring Jeanette or Frank to commiserate, but I can try to look outside myself, and think about telling some continence truths to help others feel connected.

I'm struck by how often I hear the phrase 'incontinence is common but it isn't normal', when I go exploring online. Pregnancy, vaginal delivery, menopause, hormones can increase the risks, but leaking isn't inevitable for women. It can be a moment of isolation or despair like Winterson's or a symptom like Skinner's but it isn't the natural state of things.

Can we say the same for stigma, I wonder, over those years? Is this deep-seated taboo about urine and defecation something we all *have* to live with? Surely there are areas of life where it doesn't penetrate. I go back to basics.

In sociology, stigma is seen as a process or experience, where an individual is deemed different and somehow rejected or disregarded by the society they live in, based on that difference. It has a specific meaning in medicine too: the visible element of a disease.

You don't have to probe too far to find the grubbier meanings though, the meanings that link your physical problem to a disgraceful social, personal, or ethical part of you. Making you bad and dirty. Stigma can mean a moral or physical blemish, for example. Or in even more *archaic* definitions, the mark or scar burned into the skin branding you as a slave or a criminal, perhaps arising from the idea of stigmata. A visible way of singling you out as evil, immoral or the property of others.

My difference isn't visible, except for on my worst days where I create a wet patch, but it is singled out by the society I live in as a disgusting way to be. When health and morality are conflated, that sort of ingrained horror smears everyone. But we can unpack it quite easily. It's often our human instinct to repel, ignore or heap shame on those whose misfortune suggests to us that we too may be fallible. Disability does this. Diseases like leprosy, which deforms the body and skin, do it so badly that doctors have a stigma scale listing the ways it affects the lives of sufferers. Leprosy, with its infection risks and flesh revealed, can inspire bodily disgust. Incontinence is not leprosy. Neither is depression, nor birth trauma. But in all three, the patient can feel like an untouchable, an undesirable, a pariah. That feeling isn't oversensitivity, it is borne out by how society treats people with these conditions.

I speak to staff at birth injury charity Freedom From Fistula, who help women get surgery for the horrific injuries Dr Sims was trying to solve back in the 1800s.

'We are very big on touch,' their director of operations and communications, Lois, says to me. 'Some of the women we work with haven't been touched for years. It's awful.'

Médecins Sans Frontières states that 2 million women across the globe still live with fistula, the injury that Pepys avoided. It is most common in places with poor or no obstetric care, births in remote locations, and in large numbers of 'child marriages' (as girls' smaller bodies are more likely to get hurt if forced to give birth). Even today's sufferers often face social exclusion, and the damage to a patient's mental health can be catastrophic. But though Sims' technique means it is fixable, many women can't access it. This is to do with complex aid structures, political and economic differences, but also a global refusal to engage with a dirty condition – the stigma attaching itself even to our desire to put our hands in our pockets. Taboo drains down in a wicked spiral, affecting funding and reducing opportunities to educate, heal and help. A collection of UK charities with a specific interest in incontinence for patients, including those with cancer, MS, Alzheimer's and dementia, put it starkly in 2018:

'There is a lack of funding for continence research – both historical and present – compared to funding for the search of a cure for common conditions. Limited funding, on top of the taboo attached to incontinence, makes it more difficult to attract researchers into the field.'

They added another problem too – the widespread nature of incontinence, as it affects people with different diseases and conditions, therefore treated under different specialities, means a lack of centralised action, to call for funding or policy change.

Freedom From Fistula talked to me about the weak appetite for coverage. It seems broken fannies are hard to 'sell in' to media, which is a shame as their work generates genuinely good news stories – women regaining health and status post-surgery, and finding and helping those still suffering. Post-op survivors can educate communities, challenging the belief that fistula is a curse from God rather than an accident of anatomy.

Because incontinence affects women more than men, discussions are mired in the flagrant misogyny of women's private parts being seen as dirty, as if our fannies themselves are an affront to the polite order of things. I sometimes feel the need to shout, 'Fannies are like voting intentions – private but not a secret!' It's okay to talk about both, if you want to. Nobody is forcing anyone to, but if we can't agree on this then nothing will ever change.

Women will fall into traps of utter desperation because they feel abnormal and broken, nobody will mention the psychological damage of shredded wee and poo and sex parts, girls who are forced into marriage and get fistulas because their bodies are too small to deliver babies won't even be treated with kindness. Worse, other girls, all over the bloody world, will continue to face discrimination because they can't go to school when they are on their period. ENOUGH.

And the more you look, the more you find stigma seeping in through the cracks of other disadvantages. People who have had gender alignment surgery, for example, are another marginalised group for whom continence care is necessary but sometimes falls foul of double layers of stigma and taboo.

Research has shown that trans patients 'have an increased risk for the development of micturition disorders after sex reassignment surgery' – micturition disorders being a blanket term for problems with urination – and that all patients should be given a clear idea of these risks pre-operatively, as they will need 'life-long specialized follow-up' so problems can be quickly found and rectified. This is because such surgery specifically impacts on the urological anatomy of the reassigned sex – for example, the naturally shorter female urethra being altered by phalloplasty in females who identify as trans men. Those trans men may have voiding and pelvic floor issues which they have to address, just as trans women, who are likely to retain their prostate, should remain vigilant about caring for a neo vagina and aware of potential prostate issues as they grow older. In places without the wider care structures of the NHS, or where healthcare is rationed or charged, it may be difficult to get the necessary help, or hard to ask if you have not been treated fairly before by society at large, healthcare professionals, or those in authority, as many transgender men and women have.

I feel the luck of my own privilege, as a woman whose genitals, while so frequently scrutinised in private, are not up for public debate.

But it is not all the worst kind of news, even in a world where stigma is rampant. One can argue things are at least on the up. Menstrual hygiene, period poverty and discrimination are on the agenda. Meghan Markle's list of charitable support, published for her royal wedding in 2018, highlighted this, and many women I know happily donate tampons and buy menstrual cups that automatically donate a partner cup to a woman somewhere in the world who cannot afford one or has lost her possessions in a disaster or through being displaced. We know that getting your period even on a relatively minor bad day is a total crock, and not having anything to stem the flow is stressful and unhygienic. This is a start – but has there been a trickle-down effect on continence?

I speak to Amy Peake, founder of Loving Humanity, a not-for-profit organisation that works in refugee camps helping women set up factories to make and supply sanitary products. She tells me one of the first questions she was asked when she arrived at one of the camps was, 'Will your pads work as nappies?' Aid workers and communities were desperate for continence pads for women, disabled people and the elderly, and Amy has been working to develop ways for her factories to make cost-effective adult pads (which have to be thicker) ever since.

'Sex that up with a charity ribbon if you can,' I think, though if the most quoted stats are true, and one in three women experiences incontinence in her life, then why is anyone surprised?

Amy is quiet when we talk numbers. 'They're so high,' she says, higher than she'd have guessed, and she's seen the implications.

Stigma, silence, shying away means we inadvertently treat the incontinent person badly, even at our most generous moments. Ask your local foodbanks; mine were clear that along with sanitary towels, incontinence pads are needed as they are expensive, but basic, essentials (although some people are too embarrassed to ask).

Stephanie Taylor from Kegel8, a company that makes pelvic floor exercise aids, finds it hard to get endorsements even despite increasing enlightenment about women's health.

'We have sold so many of our machines to celebrities,' she laments. 'We wish that one of the big names would champion us. Maybe one day.'

Carol, who has been talking about poo incontinence and helping me through that mess, suggests speaking to the Bowel and Bladder Foundation (BBF).

I hit a stigma stumble immediately when I read on their website that I could apply for a radar key to open disabled toilets. It would change my life. My leaky relapses, which are gradually becoming more frequent again, would be much easier and less stressful if I could use a toilet with a sink and enough room to comfortably change my clothes.

My finger hovers on the keyboard but I don't have the nerve. I've managed to control my condition publicly fairly well; I know all the tricks. Even though it definitely hampers my work and everyday life sometimes, embracing a label like 'disabled' feels too much, like I'd be blagging or overegging it. Also, I'm scared that in our austerity influenced world of disability surveillance people will challenge me using a disabled toilet even if I have a key. I'll have to explain it all, or admit it or something, and that would be too much.

The BBF staff are great, and interested in my writing and my desire to focus on the social and historical side, though they are also keen for me (well, anybody) to write about bowel issues, as even in their safe spaces it is an area of experience so ghastly that most sufferers can't lay it all out there. I want to say I've only managed to speak to them about it at all on email because I can type fast and pretend it's about somebody else, but I don't want them to be disappointed in me too.

They also put me in touch with some academics and practitioners to talk to about the wider social side of incontinence and treatment for it. They include a psychologist working with continence patients and modelling Cognitive Behavioural Therapy (CBT) group treatment on her previous work in patients with chronic pain.

I'm interested in this approach of using the mind to help because my mind is dominating so much of what is happening to me. This is one of my first interviews on the phone and as I sit in my lounge asking about her work I'm struck by how much I have to say. I break all the rules I learned in journalism (my earlier career) and burst into the narrative.

The minute we start talking, I unprofessionally let my thoughts tumble out: Are all people as ashamed? Can anyone talk about it? Does everyone else feel lonely? Where is the help if the mental collapse that accompanies incontinence is so well-known and understood?

The researcher has some interesting findings about how groups behave when talking pish.

May 2016, a lounge full of homework books and forgotten PE kits

The researcher's voice has friendly authority and she gives me more background than I expect. She's so eager to talk, and so open with her research at a large teaching hospital, that I start to suspect people working in continence care suffer from some transference of stigma themselves. Maybe nobody will actively listen to all her findings or ask about her day job talking to ladies that leak. Oh Christ, I worry. *Perhaps crucial medical research is being hampered because it is embarrassing to think about.*

Her background isn't in continence and the project emerged from an outside approach – a surgeon wondering if a psychologist may be able to help his patients with bladder symptoms deal with the fallout of that and the effect on their quality of life. Quality of life (QOL), the medical term thrown around so much it kind of melts into the background, but that has an entire index to assess which elements of a person's life their condition or illness affects the most (and how badly).

The surgeon could see that improving 'outcomes' for patients means improving the aspects of their social and wider life hampered by stigma and inconvenience. I think of the Waz Wizard and his tissues. The pause from the super-confident male GP when I referred to the spare trousers in my handbag. The quietness they offered in the face of obvious upset. They knew too.

Over the phone, I overshare my identification. The double blow, where not coping with a stigmatised condition created another one. How it cut to the core of my self-esteem.

'It's double-funk. You are failing because you are dirty, embarrassing, and socially inadequate, which is bad enough, and then you are letting the side down because you can't handle that effortlessly,' I almost wail.

The researcher understands. Her pilot used CBT to help the patients explore their own reactions and responses in order to isolate and avoid, change or challenge negative or unhelpful patterns of thinking and behaviour. The sort of thoughts that made their bladder issues dominate their life. Initially, she worried that patients might not talk in a group at all.

She explains it took a while to warm up but adds that once they started talking 'they were relieved'. I want to laugh because the word 'relieved' is so linked to the language of bladders but I don't want to interrupt as she's on a roll with another echo of my experience. Saying the women wanted to know they weren't alone, and found shared experience helped them, and once they started, it was hard to stop them talking.

I tell her how this happened when I first wrote about incontinence treatment on my blog: people talked about their current distress or sometimes incidents from years before, things they had never told anyone, not their husbands, wives, mothers, daughters. I ask if she got to the heart of the taboo and the shame.

She detours to explain the complications. When she ran CBT group sessions for patients with other disorders, for example, those in chronic pain, there was enthusiasm for involving friends and family. People with long-term chronic illness had, generally, latched onto this idea keenly, hoping that ensuring loved ones knew more about the condition, symptoms and emotional impact would help. These shared sessions helped their loved ones and carers too, and became one of the most successful elements of the treatment.

But with continence patients there was clear and immediate opposition: no enthusiasm at all. When asked if they'd like to talk about their condition with their families in a safe space, it even became clear that some of the group hadn't told their partners or families they were going to the sessions, or even about their conditions at all.

I find this shattering but predictable. The impact is enormous, and not just for the incontinent person. I know this from my little boys, who have had to traipse around to appointments and put up with my upset and preoccupations and health admin. And no doubt the effect my condition has had on my own body image, and, I dread to think about it, theirs too.

'And as for my husband,' I start, 'the impact on the lives of those you live with and love can be massive. It isn't easy to change someone else's sheets, dispose of nappies. See them reduced. Just because it isn't happening to you doesn't mean it doesn't feel rotten.'

I share what others, such as those working commercially in the continence world have told me. For example, Stephanie from Kegel8 runs an incontinence helpline, along with selling devices to help pelvic floor function. She's told me of how many marriage failures she's heard about, people who were 'absolutely over-whelmed' and felt 'their life had come to an end'. She says people often speak for ages about how they have withdrawn, 'physically and emotionally, feeling dirty and useless because they can't control a basic bodily function.'

And that's ignoring the emotional complications that make you a joy to live with, like irritation, fury, desolation, depression, desperation, self-hate, belligerence, denial.

Stephanie also says the average helpline call is 15 to 20 minutes long, and is 'usually the first time ever a woman has been honest about either wetting herself, wetting herself during lovemaking, or not feeling any sensation and feeling loose.' For her money, part of the answer is interrogating the rampant body shaming and unrealistic ideals in a media-driven society that idolises perfection, which makes everyone too ashamed to talk honestly about their own bodies.

The researcher has found similar things.

Aside from keeping the groups a closed shop, I ask her if there was anywhere that the talking and sharing didn't go?

But I already knew the answer. Sex.

'Christ,' I think, and wish I hadn't asked.

She asks if I was considering saying anything about that in the book I want to write, or my blog. Incontinent sex. The Taboo Top Trump, lording it above even depression and leakage.

'I'll think about it,' I say as we end our phone call. But I don't know if I'll dare. After all, I know something she doesn't. I have tried to talk about the effect of incontinence on my sex life before, and it didn't go very well …

Chapter 20

Sex

Some things you can't tell in chronological order, because you parcel them up and hide them until you can look them in the face with experience. Which is the case for both these episodes. I couldn't talk about them even though, or perhaps especially because, they have remained so vivid that my face still radiates embarrassment like it only happened yesterday.

Late September 2012, playing with my son while speaking to a therapist

In the therapy room, the tissues and anticipation often silence me. I can't find the beginning of my story – where did my crumbling begin? The labour ward? Motherhood? Leaking? My childish dreams? The stuckness is nearly as boring as incontinence itself.

Five years on and I'm *still* so easily rocked by any mention of my first birth that I think I might throw up with the force of my rage (or collapse completely into the cool diving pool-deep thickness of my mind, just exhale and plunge down into the cold). And I am morbidly curious about the woman I was before I went crazy, and whether she might have something fundamental to do with how I became that crazy woman. Was this always on the cards?

The thoughts tangle. Physio is going so badly I fear Lizzie will give up on me, and now I think this psychologist will decide

I am a lost cause too. It's scary. I want to be fixed and clean and normal. I just want to be at home in our gang of four and not be broken anymore.

I try to discuss this with the counsellor, an earnest man around my age, who wears linen trousers and proud open-toe sandals. He is always very encouraging. I think he can see how hard I am working to squeeze the lightness and joy out of 'loving my children and husband', clinging to it, as I hurtle along the rapids, terrified, frantically self-therapising with my blog.

I am still writing, trying to reach other people in the same boat. Searching for something. Validation? Perhaps. I'm too tired to be dishonest or coy anymore. Sometimes people ask whether I censor myself at all when I talk about incontinence in person or online (which I take as a reprimand, proof that I say too much). I do check myself, of course. Out of personal vanity and respect for the people whose lives are affected by my madness and messiness.

But I'm interested in the question. What is better, for me and for those who read what I write (or are, like this counsellor, employed to listen to me)? Do they want the whole truth or something sugar-coated? It's hard to say. I feel they expect something.

The therapist sees a loose strand and pulls. 'How do you think it affects your marriage?' he says.

And then there's a silence. All this self-reflection has been avoidance.

I nearly break the core of the earth as I shatter the silence with my withering bark of a laugh. I shouldn't have worried about the dance of show and tell – this bastard has my number after all. He's taken us to the heart of the matter.

'It's nearly ruined it,' I admit. Scared it is true.

'We can't even shag to forget about it,' I say, daringly, not adding the bitter truth: '*Well, we can shag, and we do, but I have this tiny leering voice, Mad Luce, narrating every move, making sure I will always remember I might be about to fart or piss, or worse, everywhere. And, you know, that kills the mood.*'

'But your husband still loves you, still wants to have sex with you,' says the therapist, citing our second son, sat chewing a plastic alligator, as proof. And quite without realising I am going to, I snap.

'That's worse,' I explode, knowing it could be misinterpreted as me not wanting my second baby but unable to keep it together. It has nothing to do with him, who I want and love, but it has everything to do with my brokenness. I tremble: the sudden anger is a demon, poisonous and bold, stoked up by all the people who have asked what my husband thought. A demon who's having a right laugh now, hearing someone offer this incredibly well-intentioned anodyne bullshit to me about how my husband loving me anyway makes it *all right*.

'If he still loves me and he doesn't mind sex now that I'm dirty and broken, if he doesn't care that I'm disgusting now, DOESN'T THAT JUST MEAN I'M NOTHING TO HIM BUT A FUCKING HOLE?' I counter.

The word 'hole' is too much. I've gone too far. I've shouted. And I've reduced myself to just an orifice. I'm shocked because I mean it. This is what I've become. I'm incandescent. Desolate. Nothing but a sex toy. But then there's more. There's more pent up.

'And why is everyone asking what my husband thinks? Is our sex life only to do with him, and where he can stick it? Why does nobody ask about me? Or pleasure? Or whether I can still feel anything or my scars get in the way of sex or how a prolapse changes my insides or anything?' I add. My eyes and voice prickle. I'm candid but I'm not usually so unleashed. And I can't not let the words stand because I've been wanting to shout them for months. But I can't carry on either. The outburst hangs in the room.

There's only one thing for it.

I say, 'Thank you very much,' shut my mouth, and leave.

I'm more alone than ever.

In our last session, almost a year later, I apologise to the counsellor for my shouty frankness, and tell him about when another nice professional suggested that for some people, bodily fluids in sex is a plus point, that we could just get rubber sheets and get on with it. That wasn't especially helpful advice as:

a Of course, that had occurred to me.
b If fluids were my thing – and there's no judgement; if they're yours, *cool* – I might not have complained about leaking during sex in the first place.

He says I don't need to be sorry, but I think it makes him feel better that he's not the only one who has found this minefield explosive.

I stand by my feminist concern that women's sexuality is consistently defined in terms of penetrative sex, and whether her fanny is still tight and useable for someone who wants to put something in there. It's why we joke about fannies as sleeves and buckets, and it shows a completely unoriginal and unimaginative view of sex and pleasure. I was surprised how many practitioners paused when I called this out, the idea that sex is only to do with our mangled-or-not genitals and not to do with a whole lot more.

The aggressive 'just a hole' thought badgers my brain for years. Even though this is never how my husband expresses it, and doesn't reflect anything about how we connect. In depression, my husband can't win. Nobody can.

'What's so hard to understand about not wanting to be spoiled?' I think, the few other times I talk about it, when nice normal people are kind about my state and say they are sure it doesn't stop anyone loving me, that I'm still me after all. I know they are just trying to be nice in a shitty situation. But I misinterpret it as everyone ignoring and dismissing the fact that I might want to look or feel nice. Proof that I'm too rank to deserve it.

Some advice was better; my GP, who knew us both, said she didn't get the sense my husband thought I was unloveable now. And she was right, he did still seem to want me. She said couldn't I find a way of seeing myself as attractive too, like he did? She also asked what I would think in reverse, if my husband had had a car crash a decade ago.

What's strange is how clearly and calmly I know I wouldn't give a rat's ass about damage to his body, as long as he was alive and I could tell him I loved him.

And it was through this thought that I, and we, slowly built our way back up, forcing the hardest kind of words out, learning how to talk about it, and working together on accepting the positions, props and precautions as something we just had to figure out.

My husband tried so hard. And I was so grateful for his strength, and the straightforward way he understood why I bristled when so many conversations centred around his pleasure. And I knew, really, no one was suggesting his pleasure was all — it was just that they, the few people who spoke to me about it, were just trying to find a way of talking about this that pushed beyond our ancient and primal fear of shitting the bed.

2014, when the thought of being naked in front of anybody else ever again, let alone doing anything else, has become impossible

Having a number at the bad bum clinic is taking a toll. I'm scared of everything, but mostly of my own bed. Leaking, or the fear of it, leaves me unable to speak, let alone get fruity. That's the bare awful truth of it. I feel irritated by luck and life: I wasn't asking for an epic sex life, just something 'normal', loving, fun, like I had before. I did try to trick myself out of the fear, but there's no poetry or humour or bravado that can protect you from crapping the bed during sex. Good grief.

Carol understands that I'm afraid of sex. She doesn't ask if my husband likes me or how he feels. She understands it's not his acceptance of me that's the stumbling block. It is my inability to easily accept myself, or my situation.

This seems on reflection the best basis for caring for an incontinent patient on the brink – acknowledging that their fears are rooted in a real taboo and helping them navigate their way through a new world, temporary or permanent, without acting like that's not difficult or devastating.

I don't want to disgust or embarrass my husband any *more*. I don't think he'll reject me, I think 'it' will ruin us. Take away the last shred of privacy and easiness we have. I'm not sure that's something I can bear.

Carol knows this. She listens to me talk and then holds the problem. She can't think of an answer on the spot but she resolves to dig a bit deeper. Then she rings me, a week later, to say she's spoken to a continence nurse in America and they agree that one of the bottom plugs would be safe for use during sex if I was careful. I do wonder if there is something interesting for Carol, in getting to drill down around things patients rarely bring up, but I'm too shy to ask. My intimacy chips are all spent.

'It might give you peace of mind, you know,' she says. 'After a fashion.'

It took five more years for me to find the courage to ignore the depression talking and remember that people and sex and bodies are more complex and amazing and interesting than can be imagined. And that acceptance of change isn't the same as not giving a shit about it. And clumsy references to my partner were indicative of something institutional and endemic about the way people talk about women's bodies rather than a specific slur on me.

Five years, a lot of medical interventions, more fear, and the boring, boring truth that time goes on and there comes a point for almost all situations where eventually you must work out how to make the best of what you've got. Not because it is fair, or just, or everything comes out even in the end. Because it often doesn't. But because the life you have right now is *all you have to play with*, and you can only play your best game if you remember what you've learned on the way. Any lesson, however small.

Part Five

LESSONS

Chapter 21

Feminism

I am starting to find my way, out of the worst place. To reconcile the truth: that I've been signed up, by stealth, for the incontinence long haul. That though we've thrown a lot at it, I'm still a pretty leaky thirtysomething and my poo incontinence blip might signal problems for later.

And I have started to write down my thoughts about everything (apart from the poo) to determine what, if anything, I can do to change the wet-knicker world for the better.

My blogging started because I posted an Internet rant about continence pads and all the brands touted as a solution when they are anything but. They are an aid and, for most, could and should just be a stop gap, if we stopped accepting the lie of incontinence being *inevitable* and hiding it in low-level jokes that reinforce negative stereotypes.

I call my blog 'When You Are That Woman' and become bolder as the years go by – though I find as time ticks on and I'm not quite better yet, I'm scared of disappointing readers with my lack of progress. I consider firing off emails and starting a campaign, like an even pissier Jamie Oliver, who is back then the social campaigner of his day, but a woman from Scotland beats me to it, emailing into my blog to ask if we can 'align soapboxes'. At first, I'm scared. I can speak about all this by email or online, and sometimes with friends, but I don't want people to hear the waver in my voice or to see them sneak a glance down to my crotch when I rant about pads. Sniff the air to check out my story on a sensual level.

Elaine Miller is different. As a physiotherapist, she's used to fishing around in fannies, and putting women like me at ease. As a recovered incontinent she is on a mission. Also, she's excited. Her email opens with a comment about a blog post I wrote on urodynamics.

'I've never heard a patient describe it before,' she writes, certain this silence about the other side of continence treatment is as bad for practitioners as it is for patients.

I had spent so much time trying to tease out how exactly I became *that woman*, and trying to help other women from my anonymous keyboard, but it never occurred to me that people working in the field might be interested in hearing my story too. Might benefit from hearing that there's more to patients' worry about dropping their drawers than silliness or lack of maturity.

We agree to meet and I start picking at the scab.

I track down experts, email big corporations, and revisit help-lines and charities, haranguing anyone with links to continence issues, from psychologists to physicians via product design and market research. I find loads of men and women – though mainly women – doing incredible things, from hashtag campaigns like #physioworks and #pantsnotpads to World Continence Week (WCW), which starts, in a beautiful flash of irony, *on my fucking birthday*. WCW is organised by the World Federation of Incontinence Patients (WFIP). I'm impressed by their patient-centred approach and gobsmacking stats – bladder weakness alone is more common than hay fever, for example. Their president, Mary Lynne van Poelgeest, is committed to moving global policy forward by working with others as she is clear: 'incontinence in all its forms is still plagued by stigma and taboo'.

When I ask her how many people exactly are affected, she says the best estimates are over 400 million, though full figures are hard to estimate for several reasons. Patients don't always disclose, for example, from personal shame or from not wanting to bother the doctor with something which might be dismissed as trivial. Incontinence straddles several medical disciplines (because it can be connected to so many different conditions), and so information isn't always coordinated, but also when those conditions are particularly serious, incontinence may well be affecting quality of life but it still might not be reported and recorded as it may never be at the top of the list of symptoms. Also, definitions of incontinence and bladder dysfunction vary, with some assuming leaking is normal for them due to age, sex, previous health problems. Somewhere around FOUR HUNDRED MILLION though.

All this despite the fact that the International Continence Society (ICS) – an industry-funded but a global advocate – argues that the range of treatments, procedures and surgeries available means that 'all patients' with stress incontinence 'can be successfully treated, or, at the very least, their condition significantly ameliorated'.

Product developers inventing and designing machines, pads, knickers and apps, raising awareness and helping women help themselves flood my Twitter feed week by week.

Myra Robson, a UK-based physio, creates an app with another parent from school. It's called Squeezy and helps you do your exercises. The NHS endorses it.

Mesh-injured patients set up forums and become activists. *Sling the Mesh* founder Kath Sansom's award-winning campaigning for justice is getting voices heard and applying pressure to change policy around that operation.

There are lots of examples of conversation explosions where proper care, support and treatment of incontinence is being pushed into the mainstream. There are even ad hoc multidisciplinary teams in the form of campaign groups like Pelvic Roar, who start using social media to champion best practice and promote pelvic health.

But there is still a lot of talk about how few women dare to get help.

Stephanie from Kegel8 saw this as a challenge in her sign-off response to my first email plea for allies. 'Maybe in 10 years' time, we'll have women discussing this more openly and it won't be such a social taboo,' she wrote. 'But it is up to us to drive it – to make sure that our next generation of daughters and sons understand the importance of bladder/pelvic floor health and that they have to take a proactive role in their own health. No one can help us better than we can help ourselves and our motto of "Together We'll Be Stronger" is there to help women and men know that they are not alone, and that we understand, and that we want to help.'

She was so saddened by hearing the same story on repeat: women who have told no one about their problems, hoping they will go away or get better, finding themselves housebound as young as their forties or fifties because many problems – from pelvic pain and bladder weakness to gynaecological issues and sexual dysfunction – don't spontaneously get better, and usually get worse over time.

I speak to family GP Rachel Boyce about what patients can expect at continence-related appointments so I can create the info sections at the end of this book, and also try to understand where doctors are coming from when they say things like, 'Don't get embarrassed', and what they are really trying to find out. She says the taboo around continence is analogous to the hushed silence that used to surround cancer – the original 'medical c-word'. That hush was life-threatening, and the legacy remains: patients are sometimes unable to trace back any accurate family history, especially around cancer of embarrassing parts, due to past lies told with the best intentions, to save embarrassing anyone.

Women with limited knowledge of their privates, who haven't looked or been told what is normal, are unable to spot or discuss things like skin changes, which could mean infection or even, in very rare cases, cancer.

Ignoring incontinence completely can be dangerous too, as it is a symptom not a disease. Birth injury and lax muscles like mine are only part of the story. Leaking can be a sign of neurological disease, spinal damage, prostate problems, alcoholism or mental illness.

Elaine the physiotherapist who found me through my blogging is very clear that we need to pull all these thoughts and this information together. She sets a date for us to meet. The great continence fightback has begun!

I often look back on that day and imagine what the lunchtime arthouse crowd must have made of two middle-aged women pulling increasingly ludicrous plastic moulds and pads out of a bag and screaming with laughter. Those that listened in would have been pleased to hear, I hope, my extended rant on the slippery removal of bum tampons.

Summer 2016, a busy café, Edinburgh

Pink-cheeked and dying to chat, Elaine bursts into the café with an enormous shopping bag filled with gynae goodies and giveaways. Vibrators, lube, plugs and pessaries; she's a fanny-gadget Avon lady, my broken-pussy personal shopper.

Like Carol, Elaine understands my depression response and has emailed ahead with links to the Bladder and Bowel Community, who have created a resource to address the emotional impact of incontinence, offering sensitive, sensible steps for managing the fallout. It details things like depression, sadness, fear, embarrassment. I tell Elaine their info is useful and upbeat, oozing solidarity, though I feel like something's missing.

'They forgot rage,' says Elaine. She knows.

Why are we so fearful of properly harnessing rage? I wonder. A new urogynaecologist and researcher, who I've been seeing as

I weigh up my next steps, agreed this week that incontinence is a 'feminist issue'.

'Too fucking right,' Elaine shouts. 'It is.'

Her feminism is white-hot and at the surface. I want to show her my armpit hair and talk about those strange moments in the '90s when young women, like I was then, felt we had got somewhere. Before it all went tits up and we realised we were in the midst of an anti-fem backlash, which the Internet would exacerbate, in which some young girls know even less about their body than our generation, and the visual and verbal languages of pornography dominate ideas of bodies, sex, relationships and fun.

I want to explain that I'm hopeful for the next generation, who have started to use the Internet more positively for things including self-expression. How I'm sure they might save us all, though heaven knows it isn't clear we deserve it. But do we have time to wait?

Elaine identifies her feminism as 'strident' and is prepared to lead the charge:

'Why should it be acceptable that one in three women suffer from a condition that is curable? Would men put up with it? Why are there only 11 menopause clinics in the UK? Why aren't there reproductive rights for ALL UK women? It's simple medical misogyny. The clitoris was not properly investigated as an organ until 1994. Prior to that, we knew quite a lot about the penis. 1994 … I mean, for fuck's SAKE.'

I try to remember what I was doing in 1994. Probably investigating my clitoris too.

I want to know the true effect of this taboo for women, given they are more likely to become incontinent. What is the cost of bodily oppression created by the wall of silence looming just behind the nervous joking about pishy knickers?

She reels them off, with only slight frustration – not with me, but with the world. So much of it is so obvious but we all ignore it:

- 'Women who wet themselves when they run don't run or exercise;
- 'Diseases of inactivity are responsible for one in six deaths in the UK according to the British Heart Foundation (and don't forget women are more likely than men to be physically inactive anyway);
- 'A third of women who leak are depressed because of their incontinence;
- 'Leaking in the last six weeks of your pregnancy doubles your risk of post-natal depression;
- 'Vaginal prolapse can be conservatively managed with physio – it might buy you 15 years before you need surgery. Which, given the mesh scandal, is Quite Good News. But women don't know what a prolapse is.'

I think of my own ignorance, of my anatomy, of the process of childbirth, and of the repercussions of my incontinence.

'Shit,' I say.

Elaine takes aim at sex education for leaving out menopause and gynaecological health, along with acute discomfort about airing our genitals in public and a lack of emphasis on women's rights to sexual pleasure, this creates what she calls a 'perfect storm of inhibition'. She compares pharmaceutical companies' profit margins with the cost of care and treatment. She's clear: better education, combined with giving women the tools and language to get help, could stop the economic drain.

'Tampons have been sold with detailed pictures of foofs and female anatomy for years,' she notes, sending me right back to my school bus discoveries, as she calls for clear information on packaging stating that pelvic floor exercises and physiotherapy can stop leaking.

She's passionate about thinking about women's lives as lived too – some are putting up with incontinence because 'in the intense barnstorm of parenting young children', their own wellbeing is low on the priority list. It often takes women years to get any help, even those with long-standing, socially-destructive incontinence that stops them working and ruins their sex life.

To lighten the mood, she decides to wow me with her wares, pulling a series of, quite frankly, amazing appliances and toys out of her carpetbag. We pretend they are for information, but I sense she might be guiding me towards at least considering other ways I can help myself, when I feel less beleaguered. There's new Bluetooth gizmos that work with an app and allow your health-care provider to monitor progress, see what is working and what isn't for you, how long you are exercising for, etc.

'Christ,' I say. 'No fibbing to your physio then.'

Elaine hoots.

Another is a bit of piping you insert before you clench, which leaves a straw-sized flagpole sticking out of your fanny. The angle at which the piping dangles when you've moved it inside you tells you if you are doing your pelvic floor exercises correctly. Whether it moves up or down is crudely diagnostic. And it's simple mechanics.

'Also,' Elaine adds, 'you can pretend you've got a penis.'

There are blocks that you can insert into your own urethra too. They make me wince, but I think of drunken evenings when I've wet my knickers.

'Do they work?' I ask with the marvel of a virgin looking at a vibrating egg.

'Of course,' Elaine roars, 'but they can be hard to get up, and you could end up with a UTI.' I look again. It is not tiny. I daren't tell Elaine that I'm not sure I could find my urethra any quicker than my HMRC password or birth certificate. All three, I know, are important, and have caused me quite a bit of grief, but I'm not sure I could lay my hands on any of them in an emergency.

'So many women don't know what their "normal" is,' Elaine goes on. 'And that's important for loads of reasons. How do you know if you have vulva cancer if you don't know what your vulva looks like?'

We talk about prolapses in medieval, Roman and Victorian times. Machines for wanking women. Straws made of silver for inserting slowly up your pee hole. The makeshift pessaries – from stones and paper through to the humble potato, hopefully washed, used by women with prolapses. Elaine is thrilled to hear that I've seen this in *Call the Midwife*, where a character talks about easing her prolapse symptoms – including a dragging sensation, and mild backpain – and her incontinence, with rolled-up newspaper. The show takes critical aim at the silence and embarrassment, not the tips handed down over generations, as women 'made do' with whatever was to hand.

She parades some washable pants, designed initially for heavy periods but also available for continence, including some created by TV presenter Carol Smillie. I can't decide if I'd dare to wear them, until Elaine reminds me of the chafing on your second week of being pad-tastic (two or three pads a day; another, thicker, at night).

I wince, flashing back to the horror of adult nappy rash.

'Don't forget urine burns,' says Elaine, with her radar for the rankest bits.

I think of the red-streaked skin, the rubbing, the swelling bits, the fucking nightmare of Sudocrem applied too quickly as you try to get ready for work. White grease all over your hands and your opaque tights, stains that never come out, pubes bright white. I sort of do want to forget. But we agree on almost everything else. The time has come to talk about incontinence properly and like grown-ups. Not just the physical details and the politics, but the heartbreak and history of taboo.

I can't design a new fanny plug but I can try to talk enough for other people to feel they can be heard – whether they want to talk publicly or not. To validate the desolation somehow, uncover and accept the rage and exhaustion, and provide a platform where we lose some of this crazed inhibition, condescension and stigma.

I decide to start writing again, and place myself and my story in the bigger picture.

Elaine is not just a campaigner though; she has another trick up her wizard's sleeve. Elaine wants to save the world 'one fanjo at a time', sure, but she wants to do it through the medium of stand-up comedy. She's putting the final touches to her show for the Edinburgh Fringe and, she tells me, has a dining room stacked to the rafters with vibrators to use as giveaways. Her act is packed with jokes about continence and women's health. It's designed to help solve the continence conundrum with chortles, encouraging women to feel more comfortable about their own genitals, including comfort around another 'shhh' topic, female sexual pleasure.

She thinks making women laugh, despite the dangers for those with weak pelvic floors, will help her in debunking the myths. She'll use jokes to smuggle in messages, telling her audiences what help is available, showing them pessaries don't bite, and that machines to help you squeeze no longer look like torture kits. She's ridiculing the ridicule. She has a vulva costume complete with lips, pubic hair, a clit and vajazzle, and a rubber chicken toy that she squeezes to illustrate how prolapses happen and uses as a giveaway for healthcare workers who come to her show. They come in droves, and as it is evidence-based, it counts as CPD (Continuing Professional Development) hours for them.

With a wink, she points out that she can inject plenty of sauce into the show too – as Dr Kegel pointed out back in the '40s and '50s, one of the biggest side effects of pelvic floors done properly is they can give you better orgasms.

She says she never makes fun of any situation relating to continence, birth or sexual dysfunction that isn't a situation she has been in (or could have). She isn't mining her clinical experience for pussy patsies.

'I'm the butt of the joke – incontinent people aren't,' she says clearly. She's convinced humour is a more direct and effective way to talk to women in particular about this, that it is the lifeline we need to get everyone chatting and talking, finally. She may well be right – after all, in men's health we've seen comedy campaigns like Movember, and more recently, Campaign Against Living Miserably (CALM), forcing difficult issues into the open.

I leave Elaine and walk down Princes Street, thinking of my sons, still endlessly questioning everything and fascinated by their bodies and everyone else's, having not yet learned to be ashamed of anything.

They've never asked me about my copious pads or continence, though last week in Tesco one did ask what girls have in the place where boys have a penis.

'A fanny,' I say, biting the bullet because I don't want to lose concentration and get another bollocking from the self-service machine.

'I know it's funny,' he replies. 'I said what's it called?'

Chapter 22

PMSL

When even describing your condition means saying *piss-ing yourself*, laughter is important, even if you aren't on stage trying to save the world. It can be the only way to save your sanity when you have to talk about it *endlessly* to doctors, nurses, physios, receptionists and 111 operators. When a doctor asks you to bear down as if giving birth, you have to try a joke. At least that way, when you let rip the inevitable fart, you'll be working in the right genre. I think I started to relish the spiffy one-liners as an impulse to show up something so awful.

It's why I wrote this book too, and no doubt why I swear so much and think of the most grisly descriptions: I'm trying to make you laugh so I can sneak the worst bits out into the open, in the hope some of their power will be diminished.

My incontinence confessions are vampires, or mogwai, and I'm deliberately feeding them after midnight to make them grem-lins, which are more dangerous but a far easier target. Perhaps it's the only way to show that yes, these thoughts and experi-ences are monstrous, but hell, we can fucking kill them all if we work together.

But I'm also torn.

Do endless jokes about peeing trivialise something awful? Surely it is okay to feel ashamed, rotten, and ruined if you are messing yourself in the last social disaster that people truly fear? It's the normal response.

A by-product of easy stress incontinence humour, which at least is often linked to exercise and action, is that it makes the wider issues related to continence retreat further into shadows. Athletes often laugh off a bit of damp in their running tights, which encourages a culture of silence around pelvic floor training where it is really needed, as coaches don't focus on something every high-impact sportswoman or man should be thinking about.

Specialist pelvic health physiotherapist Katharine Lough, who is also conducting research at Glasgow University, has a theory that 'oops moment' jokes make it harder to talk about prolapses too. Despite the fact prolapse may affect up to half of women in their life – it's just too icky as you can't talk about it in terms of an interruption to a good life of giggling and going for a jog, you can only use words like 'collapse', and 'falling out', and 'caving in'.

Weeing and pooing yourself *are* terrifying taboos. Tantalisingly disgusting. That's why they feature in the strongest, most controversial art as much as in pantomimes. It's why an entire generation traumatised themselves by reading *Guts*, Chuck Palahnuik's short story about a boy caught pleasuring himself on a swimming pool pump that pulls his intestines out in a long string. (Google it, you'll die.)

But even mundane gut outlet situations are difficult. Nobody wants to fart in a lift. I'd probably blush whether it was me or not. I am a sponge for embarrassment.

If I stood up during a meeting with a massive wet patch on my groin, that would be socially shaming. You can adopt the white wine trick with hot coffee, but it smarts more and ruins your clothes. Still better than the truth though, probably.

Perhaps I'm struggling because my funny bone has been collateral damage along with my perineum. Too many rude jokes at my own expense. Too much over-exposure, too much *tmi*. Or because as stand-up Hannah Gadsby points out in her trailblazing feminist show *Nanette*, jokes stop at the wrong bit of the story, the punchline comes just when you hit the horror, even if in real life the narrative of grimness and oppression is often far less comfortable to hear in full, and far longer-lasting and more widespread.

It works for Elaine to make herself the butt of her own jokes. It stops incontinent people in her audience feeling mocked and helps them feel connected. But she's the comedian in control. Maybe I'd gone too far. Used humour as a hiding place, forgetting to protect myself.

Many of the urology and pelvic health professionals I've spoken to have offered me a gentle warning about too much levity getting in the way of talking properly – the patient cracking the most jokes is always the nervous one. When humour around a condition gets too much, it can also prevent people getting help – patients across the spectrum of incontinence, not just those with post-birth injuries, will sometimes not bring up continence issues (from constipation to leakage) because they fear the doctor will be irritated at the mention of such a triviality, or think it unimportant given it is so widely dismissed.

I wonder if my 'wit' verges on the self-destructive. In their history of humour and gags, *The Naked Jape*, Jimmy Carr and Lucy Greeves describe humour as 'the last refuge of the man in trouble'. They touch on obscenity too, the humour that comes from deep dark places, and represents a delicious, often terrifying, disruption to the dedicated order of things. The indecent, unspeakable, outrageous. Probing the history of clowns, they show the seemingly modern conceit of hating them is maybe not so new. Perhaps we were always supposed to be wary of joker characters and their impulse to destruction and disorder.

Comedian and former doctor Adam Kay's *This Is Going To Hurt* took the world by storm in 2017. He'd been writing his logs and diaries over the timespan of my own descent into the darker sides of humour, so I feel a peculiar kinship when I finally read his medical memoir as I write my own. I recognise it, his snarly forensic obsession with grimness. I'm a veteran gore whore myself now. I use bald descriptions when I talk about the most humiliating, upsetting or hard-to-process things that have happened to me, even when I can tell it is going a bit far. I'm working on it now though. And I'm interested in how torn he is, between the gags and the heartbreak, the crazy mash-up of horror, venality, indifference, absurdity and joy. Perhaps that's labour ward for you – it's certainly how it felt to me the first time. Perhaps that's healthcare for you too. The price paid for looking at broken bits all day.

We all know that doctors are people too, but we expect more of them and nurses and midwives, just as we do of politicians – which is why we are so easily disappointed in any of them. And perhaps we need to bring the balance back into focus and find a way of working together, even when there is a huge trust gulf (especially after the mesh). Because if we are ever going to find a way to properly destigmatise the worst things that happen in taboo places, we must do so from both ends of the speculum.

The flipside of healthcare professionals being human is the truth that they are not innately immune to prejudice, stigma or taboo. And for continence to really be a part of a proper conversation, involving better interventions, reducing or obliviating the stranglehold shame has on patients in stopping them from seeking care, not to mention the double whammy on women – more likely to be incontinent, more likely to be a carer for someone who is incontinent – then it *all* needs to be part of a proper discussion where everything is out in the open.

Yes, most staff were pretty good to me, but are all policymakers, and funding types as cool about continence as they are about less-stigmatised illnesses and diseases? The collective fear of weakness, ageing and losing control can transcend a white coat or a budget holder's sense of deserving as easily as any other uniform or disguise. Just like it transcended me when I absorbed the shame.

Which is why the conversation needs to change; to become more human, and acknowledge all the emotions in the room, even if there isn't time to pander to them and some of them aren't very nice. And why we do need to question who and what and how we laugh about the worst things. It's also proof again that we need to start seeing the incontinent patient beyond the stereotype of the pissy old lady, the out-of-control drunk, the nervous child, the broken birther, the person in another bit of the world. Even if that means acknowledging our own feelings, from discomfort and disgust to voyeurism, fascination, pity, and indifference.

Everywhere I look, I find examples of humour that dismisses incontinent people but eventually it does something I wasn't expecting. Facing down the harsh side of humour, the gut-wrenching dizziness of standing up and raising your hand, admitting being at the bottom of the pile, the butt of the joke, it doesn't destroy me, even in my soiled underwear. It vindicates and validates all my distress: so some people DID see me as disgusting after all – I was not mad, not mad at all!

This said, I feel subdued by the hazardous game of 'truth or dare' that humorous outrage brings to the table when I talk about my own story. I'm not always helping myself or others. Especially as there's a new feeling somewhere not too far over the horizon that I can feel beginning to engulf me. A sense of ... *now what?*

My health 'journey' is, if not coming to an end, nearing a plateau. Part of me thinks a plateau would be good – there's enough change around me. My children are boys now, not babies. The eldest is approaching the twilight years of tweendom. Something bigger than a primary school joker, and closer to a teenager, or even a young man. He's stretched out, his body angular, his once round face now a heart, his almond eyes expressive, his fears and ambition all his own. The younger one too can read and write and save a penalty. He's always known his own mind, now he can express it formally. Look out, world!

Another part thinks, just like the jesters Jimmy Carr and Lucy Greeves wrote about, I need to start upsetting the applecart. That disruption is just what's needed to help me see the truth.

Maybe I can use humour as an equaliser as well as a battle cry? Elaine definitely advocates mining laughter for all its medicinal purposes. She even tells me, when we next meet up, that jokes can be diagnostic: making a female patient laugh can be very effective for physio.

'If she's giggling hard enough,' Elaine explains, 'you can feel if her pelvic floor is strong enough so she can laugh and not leak.'

Gina Barrecca, who wrote about women and comedy in *It's Not That I'm Bitter: How I Learned to Stop Worrying About Visible Panty Lines and Conquered the World*, said humour 'allows you to elevate and explore rather than denigrate or hide your feelings'. She added: 'Humour doesn't dismiss a subject, but rather, often opens that subject up for discussion, especially when the subject is one that is not considered "fit" for public discussion.'

To call out continence stereotypes throws taboo momentarily under the forensic glare of an audience. It bets on common experience of both leaking and shame and works if the pissy person is not the conduit for everyone else's disgust. That's why the laughs are explosive. As Homer Simpson says: it's funny because it's true.

I started to talk about it as much as I could; as Elaine said, making them laugh so they could hear the stories underneath the comedy. It seemed to me the stigma, and the strange conundrum that women do talk about it a bit but never more than superficially, spoke to something very deep. About our attitudes to women and sanitation in particular.

Incontinence humour thrives as the shared shrug, the one joke we women are all in on once we hit our thirties or forties or fifties. It allows unity as (mostly) middle-aged women joke about the danger of bouncy castles. Victoria Wood sold out the Royal Albert Hall with a set about shagging and ageing, in which the pay-off involved wetting herself and some glasses steaming up.

Lately, we've had Caitlin Moran's tub-thumping jokes about her weak pelvic floor used as a rallying cry for a new feminist manifesto, and her strong passion for talking about brilliant bodies forms the bedrock of *How To Be A Woman*. We've heard US TV showrunner Shonda Rhimes popularising the word 'vajayjay' and getting female orgasm chat onto prime time in *Grey's Anatomy*.

Weak bladders have a growing profile – from the raucous *Girl Trip*'s zipline scene to Australian parenting comedy series *The Letdown* via the sometimes criticised post-booze bedwetting of reality star Charlotte Crosby. Blogs, podcasts and online campaigners try daily to make women roar about the pelvic floor. Girl Guides can earn a badge about bodies and menstruation and some European countries have even started teaching about pelvic floors in classrooms. Would the teens at the back of my dusty science lab have coped with that?, I wonder.

This is all part of the post-millennium explosion in female bodily empowerment and thanks to people like Elaine saying again and again that incontinence needs to be on the agenda – as her career progresses, she's even on BBC Stories in her big old fanny costume, to destigmatise physio. CBeebies join the charge and put it on their Facebook page, to encourage the mums to do their exercises. Bring it on, I say.

But we can't become complacent. Staying too long in the shallow waters of the continence-gag does risk normalising incontinence in all but name, which won't help with awareness or those hiding a far grimmer reality. Certainly, reviewers have gotten very used to saying 'a little bit of wee came out' as the go-to risqué cover quote for comic novels or shows, but that leaves the harder truths about incontinence locked out of the mainstream.

We can build on these foundations to normalise even unfunny continence chat so women aren't afraid to speak up and get help. The damp gusset jokes are the warm-up act for the real conversation. The starting gun for a global dialogue. Because po-faced though it sounds, incontinence is more serious than a few of us worrying about farting in yoga.

Chapter 23

Men

Suddenly, it felt like the momentum wasn't just mine. I was writing and thinking about continence and women's issues a lot for sure, but I felt like I couldn't go for a piss without coming back into the kitchen to hear a radio conversation about jogging after the menopause or campaigns for better disabled toilets (too right). TV ads with smiling middle-aged women beaming at me through a haze of normalisation about how confident continence products made them. The world was demanding I woke up to, and faced down, the continence taboo, and roared at it beyond myself.

There's a name for it, beyond delusion. Seeing things everywhere is a variant on the Baader-Meinhof phenomenon, where a new or previously unknown idea is presented to you and then you look around and realise it has been there, all around you, all along. Or the zeitgeist, whereby similar ideas or thoughts emerge across culture simultaneously, as if we all share the same unconscious.

But increasingly, though there was a feminist story that I wanted to shout about, I was beginning to realise that there could be another angle I'd missed. For several years of burgeoning continence activism I have forgotten one big question: WHAT ABOUT THE MEN?

Tipping points, as we've discussed, are dangerous when you're drunk or on the brink of fury. But they can be a force for good.

When I first wrote about incontinence, one of my biggest beefs was this: why do they not make black incontinence pads? Why? When every incontinent woman who needs knicker protection for leaking that I've ever met defaults to black trousers or black skirts/dresses with black opaque tights or leggings. (As well as being super stylish, black buys you time, time you really need if you leak badly on a busy street or at work or when you are getting out of a taxi. You still feel the wind make your crotch cool if you are unlucky but from a distance it isn't obvious and you have until the smell starts to sort it out.)

As I wrote the book and pursued treatment, I found out you *can* get black incontinence pads, FOR MEN. Of course you can. Initially, I was furious. Why do men get practical black inserts, which don't give a glowy white bulge, while women are offered papery monstrosities that look like deformed nappies, or worse, flowery pants that my grandmother would have deemed unfashionable?

What gives? I thought, writing to Tena's mother company SCA to ask. But no response was forthcoming.

It seemed male incontinence was getting far more serious treat-ment than women's. I genuinely found forums where men were allowed to ask a doctor a question, while women were directed to a nurse, or physio. It seemed women were sent to chat amongst themselves while men were treated as serious patients.

And even when this updated as time went on, women's incon-tinence products were still framed as a way of coping without the worry of unexpected leaks and the commensurate social anxiety, while men were encouraged to decisively move on from an outra-geous state and 'take back control' of their lives.

For fuck's sake, I thought. *Men get bloody everything. Even to feel like incontinence is not a natural part of their life's trajectory.*

By 2017 I am at peak ranty-pants. My feminism is unleashed. I am about to hit 40 and, like the memes say so eloquently, my garden of fucks has grown barren. My temptation is to grump on about how much money is spent on male incontinence product development and marketing and the newspaper articles I read fawning about how brave it is for anyone to tackle it. And yet I am still keen to write about men because I have a sneaking suspicion that far from getting the best deal ever, their incontinence is tainted with the same stigma as women's, only inverted.

I get a huge response in early 2018 for my first widely-shared published piece on becoming incontinent. Senior women, journalists writing about women's health who have never acknowledged their own issues, charities and campaigners contact me, including many in private DMs talking about how they'd never felt able to talk before. But I also hear from men: one tweets to thank me for mentioning them in what is often seen as women's shameful domain. He says men felt ignored in some of the incontinence discussion and awareness raising. Their experience is just as baldly awful, just as upsetting and socially wired for shame and contains the same drudgy nonsense – like choosing between strong pads or pants that will cause an unsightly lump in the silhouette of your trousers, or something more svelte that may not catch enough wee or poo to keep you dry in public. It strikes me that perhaps our long history of patriarchal cultural oppression, and having our bodily functions stigmatised, has given women the advantage in this arena.

The landscape of continence is stacked in a way that's hard for men to navigate. Though women tend to become incontinent gradually, by the time they do they are entirely used to their state of oppression and can cope with the trappings. Everyone who menstruates has had to become a cotton product Ninja, well-practised in slipping a rustling pad into a cardigan pocket and running to the loo, without alerting anyone. Men who become incontinent are thrust into a complex new world without even a tampon leaflet to help them.

Women often find a supply of sanitary towels and pads in their shared toilets, and pretty much all ladies loos have a bin. These seem like little things, but incontinent men must feel like first-period me. Dismayed to find pads and bum tampons wriggle out of their wrappers like snakes shedding their skin, and get lost at the bottom of your work bag (if you even have a bag which many men don't). Panicked when there's nowhere to throw things away. No bin is also a perennial nightmare for those using men's toilets who need to dispose of stoma bags.

It underscores the feminist point – just because something aggravating for your gender has become so commonplace you've forgotten it is learned doesn't mean it is natural. It doesn't have to be the state of things that women sort out and put up with body mess and discomfort. You are just used to it. Men aren't – look at how many of them are totally prepared to piss up the side of a public building because they haven't walked past a toilet in 20 seconds.

Men who become incontinent haven't spent a good few afternoons picking through a snowstorm in their pubes after their period started unexpectedly at Aunty Jean's and they had to resort to a loo roll bung. Most men haven't had to consider how to trial a new form of protection, like a menstrual cup, while ensuring they will be near places where the sink and the toilet are in the same room, to save having to wash bloody hands in the flush, and creating a *Dexter*-style crime scene.

They have none of this. But they do often have to queue for the private part of their public loo. Where can they put their soiled pants? How long will it take them to remember to use the wrapping from the replacement pad to wrap up the old one, or master the art of pant fodder origami?

Becoming incontinent was terrible, but I didn't have to take a crash course in handling sanitary products at the same time. Further, women are sounding out the first rumbles of our massive communal body roar. We are learning to start showing our bits and become less afraid. Men are at the starting block with incontinence after centuries of being in the front seat for everything else apart from emotional issues.

For men, the strong link with ageing is also an issue. Prostates can enlarge as you grow older – and a change in the size of your prostate, which is around the size of a walnut normally and lives under the bladder, can cause symptoms which range from the irritating to the alarming. They can slow down or stop the flow of your wee, making it dribble or making you need to pass urine more often or even make your wee contain blood too. It may go hand in hand with erectile problems for some. But many men with prostate problems now are of a silver-surfing modern generation; they do not feel old enough to be like their great uncle Wilf who always needed a widdle, even though a family tree would probably show their ancestors' issues kicked in at the same age. Along with the psychological and physical impact of leaking, frequency can result in sleep deprivation too.

Men's public health is fascinating, but it has its own male-centric taboos to face down – like a propensity to be crude or brave, and the stigma around male talk of emotions and depression. But being controlled by wee is just as depressing for those men who suddenly find they dribble in their Y-fronts, always need a pee and are exhausted from being up and down all night.

Also, men's incontinence is often a result of surgery for prostate cancer, or in younger men, relating to difficult diseases or injuries. It starts in the context of major health trauma. Poor bladder or bowel control comes on top of horrible surgery, disease or prognosis. Though even men hitting their fifties and sixties without cancer in their prostate will often start experiencing emptying issues.

In the UK, as elsewhere, this will become increasingly common as men live longer, and expect and anticipate an active life. Larger elderly populations mean more men managing incontinence or other urinary issues. No wonder products aimed at men are a massive area of investment and women's health physios are now called pelvic health physios (this also means they are more inclusive, allowing all patients to get the care they need).

Also, there's something else. As I immerse myself in self-reflection and think about the origins of all this taboo and stigma, I do ruminate on my lack of preparedness more than once. I contact antenatal teachers, both my own and friends who have become them. I want to know, 'Are many women as stupidly ill-prepared as I was?' I feel sheepish as I ask around, but I get lots of similar responses.

'Women are massively unprepared,' says one, an old friend who's now a birth advocate and campaigner. We talk online about my early memories and she shares the pictures and diagrams she uses to ready women for what their body may go through, pictures designed to help women she teaches make their own best, consenting choices about birth. One highlights a female pelvic floor before and after pregnancy (see diagrams opposite).

'God,' I think, marvelling at the stretch and how unlikely it seems that any, let alone so many, women emerge fairly unscathed, and not knowing quite whether I'm pleased or not that I'd never seen that so starkly.

We rant about how maternal health is not prioritised, how our bodies, especially our vaginas, are discussed and derided, and how hard it can be to find clear, unbiased evidence and advice to make relevant decisions about any of it.

'We ought to live in a society that prepares us all our lives – which we would if there was less taboo,' she says.

She shows me another diagram that is so unfamiliar I wonder if I studied the wrong mammal at school. It is like a perverse, flayed apple (see diagram on page 248).

'What is *that*?' I ask.

'It is a man's pelvic floor,' she types.

Female Pelvic Floor Anatomy

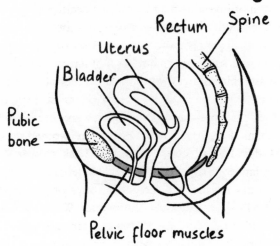

Rectum

Spine

Uterus

Bladder

Pubic bone

Pelvic floor muscles

Normal

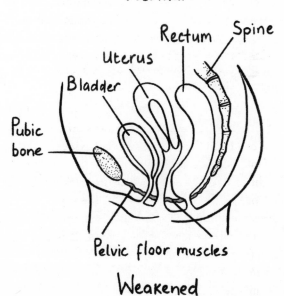

Rectum

Spine

Uterus

Bladder

Pubic bone

Pelvic floor muscles

Weakened

Male Pelvic Floor Anatomy Internal View

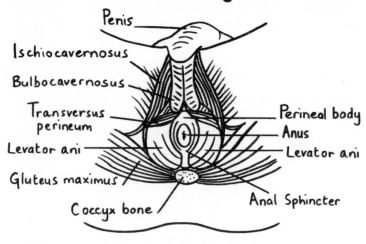

Penis

Ischiocavernosus

Bulbocavernosus

Transversus perineum

Levator ani

Gluteus maximus

Coccyx bone

Perineal body

Anus

Levator ani

Anal Sphincter

I'm intrigued. It turns out she shows it to her classes too, as a public service, because many men don't realise they even have one.

'Blimey,' I think.

'Do the men appreciate that new knowledge?'

'They are WELL uncomfortable,' she confirms.

I'll bet, I think. Perhaps we are all hindered in getting help by a lack of anatomy basics.

So, men have a pelvic floor too, they just haven't been hectored into exercising it one way or another all their lives. Even though big risks to the male pelvic floor include things lots of men do – like jobs that involve heavy lifting, and playing contact sport.

I ask Elaine how men can do their pelvic floors, and she says, with only a hint of relish, they must imagine they are stuck in a tank filling up with icy-cold water, and try to lift their balls up to avoid the sting. I have yet to meet a single man who knew this. I can imagine it will produce the same startled faraway gaze that women have been perfecting for years at traffic lights as they squeeze.

Stephanie concurs, noting people in her business estimate that male pelvic floor health is at least 10 years behind women's, where messages about exercising and some forward-thinking practitioners are starting to make the conversations more likely. Men have nothing, not even the legacy of Victoria Wood talking about the improbability of clenching in public.

'We are trying though!' Stephanie says. 'And the pad manufacturers are advertising in men's toilets now.'

She sees her role as encouraging and raising awareness of pelvic issues for men too, to keep the prostate healthy and to help with leaks and weak flow.

I have a sudden thought.

She has spoken to me about testing equipment herself and with volunteers, making sure her tools work properly for women. Does she have a male panel too? She demurs. Yes, she has male volunteers, but she can use her own bottom too even if she can't replicate stimulation for erectile issues.

Which I guess is the kind of answer I deserve. Maybe it has even shocked me out of my squeamishness forever.

Chapter 24

Medics

The trouble is, despite these thoughts, these crusades, these attempts to work out what I think about my incontinence, my body is still not quite right. My medical journey has been on hiatus as I learned to be a bit more myself again, but it still isn't over and despite my public face of cross crusading optimism, I know I am getting worse again. And I need to make a decision – live with my continence woes escalating, or see if we can find another solution.

A strange event, another Christmas party, though thankfully not one where I wet myself completely, is the catalyst (along with my impending fifth decade) that sets me thinking about how I can forge forwards into the incontinence twilight and also, perhaps, understand the medical world I've been living in for almost a decade just a little bit better.

December 2015, another Christmas party

I am sitting next to a midwife. I try not to talk about my births anymore, but I want to look engaged. I ask what her favourite bit of the job is and she tells me: suturing.

'Why?' I ask.

She goes into a reverie. For her, it is the challenge, fitting and sewing the itty-bitty pieces back together, a soft-tissue jigsaw of genuine importance. She has your sex life and future in her hands and must work quickly with her curved needle to unravel all the damage and ensure it is not too loose, not too tight, all the right parts are stuck back together, that no bit of your intimate self, functional or presentational, is lost. She tells it like a bedtime story, her wonder is infectious as she acts it out. You can see she's thinking of her pride and satisfaction in the image of all the shredded fannies she's ever cleaned and saved, and that she's probably projecting some of them in her mind's eye as she describes it.

Other party guests look slightly nauseous over their chocolate torte, but I'm entranced.

I now have years of practice at small talk and jokes with hands exploring my pelvic floor. And I've been so lucky meeting so many medical people, healthcare workers and other experts committed to destigmatising their world and willing to hear me when I point out the contradictions or absurdities of some of their stock phrases. Like 'Don't be embarrassed' or 'We've seen it all before' or even, when you have no idea how you can possibly be saved and no medical degree, 'How can we help you?'

But I've never thought about the viewpoints in opposite. The worst day of one person's life, a chance for the other to shine. For one, a traumatic life-changing injury, for the other, a fascinating and complex puzzle, an opportunity.

The healthcare community seems desperate for the stigma to be diminished, but they can't all be immune from embarrassment and all the other humiliating emotions themselves, can they? We want our physicians and nurses to empathise with us and be kind – but we all know really that it is just as important that they don't overidentify with the patient. These are blurred lines for all of us.

When I take part in a study on pessaries, for example, which aims to identify research areas by taking concerns from both patients and clinicians, the organisers confess that in early surveys they asked participants to identify as one or the other, forgetting that many people might be both. One in three is a big statistic.

Just because you are a nurse, or physio, or surgeon doesn't mean you'll automatically avoid the problems you treat.

I decide to try and get more help – even if a second run at surgery is not an easy sell to myself.

I am fed up of being a patient, even if I am still not dry. I even avoid the so-called sabotaging behaviours common in women who don't respond to treatment. I am good, I do my exercises every day, and I don't wear pads 'just in case', all things which may stop me being mindful of my condition, but still I leak.

But as apps start to tell everyone around me to exercise gratitude, I realise part of gratitude, for me, isn't putting up and shutting up, but going for another roll of the dice. Yes, I am quite tired of it all, but no, I will not give up just because my first op wasn't 100 per cent successful.

I decide to go and ask for help again, back in Urogynaecology.

September 2016, same large teaching hospital, new doctor with new ideas

My new doctor is another member of the Waz Wizard's team. He does not seem tired even though he has just reviewed my extensive files, which must be an exercise in drudge. He's not perturbed though. He's disconcertingly excited and bursting with ideas. He understands my disappointment that my suspension op didn't work completely, though he looks at me with astonishment when I say I'm worried I've failed or disappointed the Waz Wizard. This sort of reflection, this focus on inadequacy, doesn't play in his world of fixing.

He suggests a 'Tension-free vaginal tape' (TVT) operation aka the mesh surgery, as I am a reasonable candidate, but he's aware the operation is not a neutral suggestion given the reported issues for some patients and says I should take my time and think about it thoroughly.

As we now know, the mesh scandal remains a live issue. And there's been updated guidance since my meeting with the surgeon. By the time I'd finished this book NICE had put a high-vigilance restriction period in place for the use of vaginal mesh to treat stress urinary incontinence or pelvic organ prolapse, with NHS Improvement and NHS England sending a letter outlining the terms to CEOs and medical directors of UK trusts. That meant effectively no surgical operations involving mesh should have taken place during this period unless a particular patient's circumstances met a number of very specific conditions.

If the pause is lifted, surgical options involving mesh can be offered again, but since April 2019 the NICE guidelines on urinary incontinence or pelvic organ prolapse state non-surgical options should be considered before any other type of treatment. They also emphasise giving patients clear information about the choices available, and the risks of surgical interventions.

When I think about having the op, friends email me newspaper articles about the risks and horror stories. I hear of a leaky birth injury warrior from back in my forum days who had the op and now needs a walking stick. Another friend confesses she now lives with a clear fear that her mesh – once a huge salvation – may go wrong at any moment. 'It has worked well, *so far,*' she says. There are many of these stories that still need to be heard.

They are not my story but the potential complications pose a quandary for me too. My first operation didn't completely stop my incontinence, but it didn't leave me more broken. I have to try to work out whether the risk of complications is one I am prepared to swallow for the promised Holy Grail: a life without leaking.

The doctor doesn't hide any risks from me. He gives me pages and pages of studies to read. This puts me in a far better position than many women who had the mesh op, though it doesn't make things clear – I am a patient, and though I'm smart enough, I lack the skills or vocabulary to compare the studies properly.

This medical data is impossible to digest. Some of the trials are on older women than me, for example, and there seem to be

many different types of mesh. I don't know if that makes a difference. And it isn't always clear if the surgery was the same, or how
'success' was defined.

By now, even cursory Googling pulls up a wealth of stories
about lawsuits and injured women, and medics I speak to outside
my own case do talk about the mess it has left their discipline in.
I have a lot to think about.

Writing about the mesh now is hard. All my sympathy is for the
patients whose lives were ruined, of course. And I have no sympathy for surgeons if they lied, or any number crunchers selectively
muting patient voices. Or for doctors who fudged their answers
or outright lied when women asked if the mesh they'd read about
was being used on them.

I do have broader sympathy, though, for a community witness-
ing the collapse of a revolutionary surgery. One physio I meet
says she saw a presentation from a TVT pioneer years ago when
it was still seen as a radical solution. I ask her what he was like.
Her answer: humble. Humbled by being involved in something
transformative, perhaps because like surgeons of the past, desperate to solve the worst birth injuries and traumas, he was thrilled
to have found an easy fix for such a horrid problem that wouldn't
need to be rationed.

The mesh was seen as the ultimate magic bullet, the answer to a
medical issue as old as time. Perhaps it was just too hard to resist the
dream that a super-quick slice and a nifty plastic hammock would
do the trick and end millennia of invention with an easy cure.

I guess I was saved by timing *twice* – I wasn't offered the
mesh the first time because I was too young, but by winter 2016,
there was more research and experience which meant I was
older, wiser, and more bolshy. I was given the evidence to read
about all my operations, and when I wobbled over the mesh, the
surgeon offered me the option to have urologists build a sling
from my own tissue.

Lucky as I was, it felt for a while that my capacity for making, or even seeing, choices open to me and recognising where I may have agency for changing anything myself was fused shut. I was paralysed, and not just by having such a well-known unmentionable condition, but by now having to weigh up years of medical evidence which seemed to pitch women's testimony against the medical world's definition of a 'successful' operation, as if these should always be in opposition.

In response to powerlessness we often assert our desire for choices, but when the chips are down, choices are sometimes the worst thing of all. Obstacles for us to pick a careful route between, rather than a comfort.

December 2016–April 2017, hospital, again

I'm a regular now. The surgeon has sent me so much information I feel swamped. And a bit like I've been given all the responsibility, because medicine went wrong. I can no more weigh up the medical evidence written for journals, and with such widely different parameters, than a child can drive a car.

My husband has sent some questions ahead of our latest appointment – about specific types of surgical tape used and study composition, but even if this doctor knows the answers, we realise that we won't know what to do with the information.

The list of risks outlined to us include:

- mesh erosion (the mesh cutting into tissues, nerves, organs through vaginal walls);
- nerve damage;
- punctured bladder;
- UTIs;
- dyspareunia (difficult or painful sex).

I become fixated on one of the smaller risks. One based in my irrational but still enormous fear of the bodily. With sling ops, there is also a small chance of being left having to use a catheter to empty yourself, permanently. Just the thought makes my chest tighten. What if there's a nuclear war and I survive but run out of supplies? What if I drop my last one down the toilet when I'm camping and my bladder explodes? What if I am shit at it and stick a straw up the wrong hole?

Unlike one doctor who remarks that I am particularly 'hung up' on detail, this man takes a deep breath and makes a promise. He sends us home to think some more, with his solemn oath that if I elect to do anything that risks this outcome, now or in the future, he will have me into clinic and show me how to put in and use a catheter. He assures me, as is later corroborated when I meet people who do it, that for many there's something very straight-forward and empowering in self-catheterisation as it gives you an element of control you didn't have previously.

He treats my increasingly skittish caution (which must be aggravating) with sympathy and wry observation, telling me he understands: 'It's not like picking a curry.'

'No,' I think, visions of a scalpel near my vagina dancing in my head. 'No, it is not.'

We go home and I think some more. But the more I hear about the mesh, the more I think I can't risk it. My mobility is already affected by arthritis, and my experience of chronic pelvic pain and SPD was too much. I will do anything to avoid being that woman again.

The surgeon is not cross when we return and confess we have decided it sounds too invasive. Somehow, I am still afraid he will admonish me.

Maybe he's nicer than them, or less stressed, or just happy, as he has another trick up his sleeve, another option. He starts talk-ing about a new technique that involves injecting bulking agent into my bladder neck (no, I don't know either, even after he shows me a video on his phone of him squirting it) and I Google the astonishing syringe fandangos used to insert it. The theory is it will stop things waggling and get me what I realise I have been chasing for years now – a ceasefire in the wretched knicker wars. Some dry time. Perhaps brief. Perhaps not permanent. Nothing more than that.

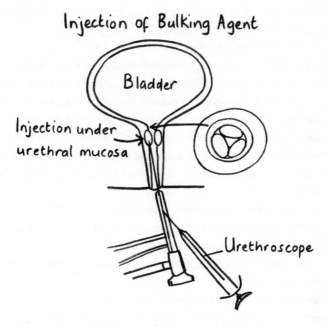

It would be something.

There isn't a lot of research into the injections, which makes me wary, but the evidence there is seems to suggest far fewer risks than the mesh. And there may be new options in the future if it doesn't work.

The surgeon is injecting some humour into the proceedings too, along with his Bulkamid hydrogel. He has a sly and witty turn of phrase, and a love of puns, which leaves me nervous and slightly thrilled about what might come next every time he opens his mouth. He's described me, not without a tone of admiration, as a 'prolific pee-er' already, and concludes with a sales pitch for these injections that are, he smiles, 'just what the doctor ordered'. I feel like he might have thrust both thumbs at his chest, music hall style, or pulled off his *CSI* sunglasses, when he said that, but I could be imagining it. He also appears to do the British Sign Language sign for 'vagina' with both hands when he's describing where he will be going to correct the 'waggle' of my urethra. But again, he might just be subconsciously checking I know what the words mean.

If the Waz Wizard is Harry Potter, this guy is one of Ron Weasley's twin brothers. But though he's a joker, he's treated me like an adult when it counts. I even forgive him for signing me up for another urodynamics test as if it was nothing.

I agree to it, but I have a full-on wobble when I find out it is on a weekend. I feel pathetic but I am upset because I know Carol won't be there. I email like an idiot, but she replies kindly to say, 'You can do it, Luce.'

Her faith in me is as important as my faith in myself – and she's right. The test is fine. There are only three staff, one to chaperone while two male imaging specialists get to work. One walks me to the wet room and asks, out of habit, have I had this test before?

'Yes,' I reply, and he stops in his tracks.

'And you came back?' he says. 'You're brave.'

I am on course for a far higher score today, I think. Maybe I'm A* material after all.

We prove I still leak and they leave the room for me to empty myself at the end, for privacy. It's quite splashy still, but I appreciate the thought. They also tell me about one hospital where these tests are done on the top floor, the building so high it's safe to leave the curtains open so the pisser can see a relaxing view of the countryside.

'Thank God for deep down corridors,' I think. 'Nobody needs to see this show.'

In April, we go for broke, and I rock up for a second operation. It's Easter, and sunny, and even though it needs a general anaesthetic, I've been assured, and reassured, that this is a simple day surgery.

I do well until I get to the shiniest corridors in the surgical wing. I'm trying to be brave. I don't want fear to spread like wild-fire. But there's something about the bright lights and my gown that blows air on the embers as I walk towards theatre.

I want my husband, my sisters, my parents to walk me to the door. Our doula to keep me calm. Or even, I realise, now, I'd like my little boys to hold my hands, to guide me gently to the theatre and squeeze my fingers extra tight because they know I don't really want to go. They can't though, because they are out with friends trampolining, and anyway, the corridor is sterile. I walk alone, see the bed and climb on, hoping I've not flashed too much flesh. My eyes sting and I wonder if I should reconsider. Then it happens.

'Luce,' says a familiar voice from somewhere I can't see because I'm flat on my back, or 'supine' as I now know the gynaecologists like to say.

A head appears over mine. It's the Waz Wizard. He's seen my name on the board and come to say hello. All these years later and we're back, him looming over me, polite and charged up, exuding his enthusiasm about fixing women like me. He's been in on discussions about me and he thinks it is a good idea from his younger colleague. We small talk about the procedure.

I can't remember how to pronounce Bulkamid – it's the Latin words all over again – so I go for simplicity and say 'thank you'. And then because I'm a lunatic, and nervous, I add: 'Wish me luck.'

He smiles. And does wish me luck. I don't need to crack a crass joke or save face. Because I am sincerely grateful and there's nothing else to say. Touched that he remembered my name, I do feel emotional. I want him and Carol and all of them to know that I remember theirs, their names, and kindnesses to me when I saw myself as nothing but a pissy woman, too young for their clinic, disgusting and unhelpable.

And that I will always be grateful for their commitment to helping me. And for this simple gift of a friendly face and a familiar voice, full of hope before the lights went out. Whatever the meaning of this brief moment from his point of view, he has helped me. I slide easy into the anaesthetic this time. Fingers crossed, legs open.

Chapter 25

Coping

Coping with incontinence is no picnic. There are some women and men for whom, it turns out, the answer is: tie a cardigan around your waist, avoid trampolines and hope no one notices the faint whiff every now and again. More power to their elbow; nobody has to accept shame just because it is there.

When I found myself standing on a hill, after that first doctor told me I had a prolapse and a proper problem that went beyond an occasional blip, I did not have such easy resolve. I was devastated, scared, incredulous, lonely and ashamed. But mostly, I was angry.

I didn't know how I was supposed to react. People kept telling me not to be embarrassed, usually as they washed my pee off their hands before talking me through another load of exercises or treatments or grim prognoses. But how do you move on with your life when you're still only one step away from being stitched up? How can you enter a healthcare world connected with embarrassing and disgusting things, and come out of it, pull your damp pants on and head back to the office with a selfie-ready smile on your face that says: 'I'm winning at life and this mum business, and I'm totally fine'?

And how do you find the right treatment and help, or know when you must move on to the next phase of acceptance and lifestyle changes? It is hard enough even when you decide you are going to try to get help. Bar none, every healthcare professional

I spoke to was clear – help is out there, both for cure, and for finding a way to live with problems that cannot be cured completely.
They were all sensitive to the enormous stigma but entirely
committed to making sure I didn't feel stupid or rank if I asked
them for help.

But that is a wider context. Incontinence is shameful and taboo
and a private prison if you don't have help, free or accessible
healthcare, or the brass balls to shout about it. Incontinence *is*
a perfect storm. It is upsetting, abnormal, hilarious, silly, messy,
stinky, undertreated, treatable, dirty, strange, and many other
things. As a condition, it hides in the open, pretending it is a simple
problem easily talked about and solved. The 'simples' attitude is
a millpond though, an illusion. There's a deadly undercurrent of
taboo just beneath the surface. We know this, or millions more
people would get help with it.

If you are leaky, for whatever reason, I can't tell you how you
should react or what you should do. I've explained how I did.
Hopefully, you can make a better fist of it than that! But please,
if you can manage it, try to get help. And whether you do or not,
remember you aren't a lunatic if you find it not ideal to leak.

Asking how anyone is supposed to respond is a trick question. When it comes down to brass tacks, I don't have a save-all
answer. Instead, I have two rude stories to send you on your way.

In my healthcare life I am an apologiser and a joker. My default
response to being in hospital for anything is forthright, if defensive, bold talk, or embarrassment. When I get over that, I defer
to authority, even when I disagree with it, for as long as I can
(or, as you've read, retreat into trauma and madness). Sometimes
that works, very occasionally it results in me exploding a little,
either huffily – chucking my fury and upset out at whomever isn't
listening to me – or self-deprecatingly, blaming myself for the
entire situation and crying in a toilet.

Over time, I've taken many approaches. I've denied my condition, owned my shame, overshared and made jokes of it. I've also

learned to arm myself with advice and find tactics for the most embarrassing and horrid appointments. I've printed out lists of questions, looked up statistics, taken someone with me to ask the questions that I daren't, and practised what I was going to say and ask for in front of a mirror. I've even drafted questions on my phone and thrust it into the palms of a lovely male GP who was startled at my honesty, but glad I'd told him my worries in electronic form at least. There are loads of ways to talk about taboo things. You can and will find one if you need one. Promise. I've even put some at the end of this book.

This book has been my story, but for the sake of rounded advice and understanding, I'd like you to meet two people who had different ideas about medical help for something desperately embarrassing. Let's call them Carrot Woman and Pear Woman. It seems to me that in our crazy and complex world they are in some way HEROIC ROLE MODELS for us all.

My friend knows a doctor. During his training, he did a stint working in emergency medicine. A bright young thing, he was eager to help a woman in pain. He examined her thoroughly and quickly found the problem. She had a carrot inserted so far up her vagina it had got stuck.

He asked pleasantly: 'It looks like you have a carrot stuck in your vagina. Do you know how it got there?'

She replied: 'I know I've got a carrot stuck up my fucking vagina. How it got there is irrelevant. Take it out.'

Boom.

Heroic.

I want to be Carrot Woman, for the rest of my life.

Next time a doctor asks me to drop my knickers, unless it's George Clooney in *ER* c.1994, I'll say: 'I know it's a mess, but this is your problem now. I'm one of your ladies. You sort it out.'

But human beings are complicated. And that isn't the only way to handle a stressful fanny situation, as it turns out. When I told this story to my sisters, resolving to change my tack and improve my confidence as a patient, they topped it.

For they also know someone, this time a nurse in A&E. This nurse also met a woman complaining of pain and vaginal discharge. She examined her and quickly saw the problem: The patient had a mouldy pear stuck up her vagina. Yup. A mouldy pear. Squishy.

She and the doctor tried to explain to the woman that she had a mouldy pear stuck up her vagina. But though it was clear she did know about the pear, the patient, or client, interrupted them and said: 'No, I don't. I don't know what you are talking about.'

Throughout their assurances, questions, and the pear's removal she kept it up (her provocative denial, not the fruit). As the docs grabbed and cleaned up the slimy culprit and gave her antibiotics, she went on the attack, maintaining nothing so embarrassing or weird could possibly be happening to her, and perhaps the medics should look to their own dirty minds. I like to imagine it going like this:

'That's disgusting! Who would do that? I don't even *like* pears. And besides, why would *anyone* put a pear up their vagina?' I like to see her, sideways looking to camera, unwilling to discuss it as she held her line, like a chocolate-covered two-year-old staring at an empty Easter egg wrapper and shouting with indignation: 'It wasn't me.' And then with a final flourish shouting something like: 'What is it about YOU that makes you assume this is all about sex?'

There is such a deliciously fruity kernel of truth at play in both these stories. Shame can take many guises. You don't have to be an apologist for having a rank thing go wrong with your body. You could be a Carrot, or a Pear.

I'm not an expert in psychology or therapy. I honestly don't know how to reframe anything beyond common sense. Like trying to be as kind to yourself as you would be to others, and remembering that bodies are bodies, and most people are quite nice and human about most things. And that if you are in a cultural or institutional or any other setting where your treatable problem is stigmatised, then there is still help out there for you, in other places where it isn't as stigmatised, like healthcare settings, new friendships or even online forums.

June 2017, sunny city centre, the morning of my 40th birthday party

I'm planning a massive party to celebrate this fucking decade being over. All the talk of ageing is making me thoughtful, so on the way to buy every nearly-40-year-old's best friend, a make-up session at a glitzy shop with the promise of luminous skin and a fuck-the-world red lipstick, I impulsively duck into a pub, pull into a booth and start to reflect on the changes coming, and those that have been.

I am not madly depressed. I don't have to guzzle the booze or be sick with Mad Luce ranting in my ears. And my appointment is an hour away. I can just sit. Thanks to the bulking agent, I can handle one glass without getting leaky these days, and I'll decide this evening whether to wear pads for my bash depending on how it feels. Sitting in the quiet of the bar, all pale wood and shiny fittings, I am ready to ask the questions.

'How far,' I think, 'have I actually come?'

I have time. Do I dare take a last look at who I was before all this shiz started? It's almost a decade to the day since a fat-faced, furious, pregnant me was raging that she'd be the only one unable to drink at her 30th but super excited about what was to come, and it feels right that I should dust her off one last time for prosperity before I hit a new decade.

I have to scroll through my phone. But there she is, at the beginning of social media, posing with her bump. I think of the day I did my test, and the conspiratorial texts between her and her husband:

'I'm pregnant.'

'Tee hee.'

She had to practically put both hands over her mouth not to tell everyone she met she was going to have a baby.

It is tempting to ridicule her – standing face open to the world, still convinced she'll write a book and have time to wash her long, long brown hair on maternity leave – and blame her credulous innocence for the mental collapse, and perhaps the physical one too. If only she'd learned more about her pelvic floor. But as the years drive on, I don't want to. In fact, I want to cling to the memory of her for a little bit longer.

As if in a movie, a pregnant woman and her friend walk into the pub. I catch the echo of my thoughts in this gloriously bent-out-of-shape stranger, laughing with her friend. Proud belly in a stripy top, John Lewis wish-list on her iPad, presumably no fucking idea what will come next.

Like the world, I project myself freely onto her pregnant self.

And then I feel kind. Kind to her and kind to me. That lovely, would-be novelist me, with all that imaginary time on her hands between breastfeeds and nappy changes. She was nuts and off the mark. And yet? I think she reflects a certain sort of strong ambition and complete naivety and, despite her ignorance, I'd like to get a bit of her unworldly wonder back.

She's a beacon. Like this lady on the table next to me, sipping her orange juice and giggling. She represents a driving force, an idea of me from the days 'before'. Before I had children, or incontinence, or a form of PND or PTSD or whatever the final diagnosis was, all as a result of a dreadful labour and difficult health narrative. The days when I was a different, happier woman, who wanted a baby, and held the, not unreasonable, hope it wouldn't be terrible, who had never had a difficult diagnosis of any kind and who had remained successfully potty-trained for around 27 years.

I want to hold onto her tightly and feel her thrills of ignorance, and somehow make her bottle it. One of life's meanest tricks when things are tough, when a joyous moment is superseded by dreadful luck or horrid events, is not just the fact that bad things have happened, but that when they do, it can obscure all the hope and lust for life and eye-sparkle that was there before. How sad to be robbed of both the good event itself and the nice feeling of the anticipation for the good thing that never happened (but should have done).

For years, it wasn't soothing to be reminded. The sight of a pregnant woman would have made me leave my table, or neck my drink and order a bottle, but today I don't.

Pregnant women scared me, made me feel tearful. I was worried I'd ruin them if I told them anything true about my post-birth life. Like those old wives' tales about pregnancies being jeopardised if women so much as looked on anything gruesome or deformed.

I thought they'd smell my failure on me, along with the *eau de pis*. Now I feel mostly hopeful as I cry looking at my phone, and she no doubt thinks I'm a sad old hag, drunk on a Saturday morning. Really though, I'm kind of happy. I'm hopeful she and all the other pregnant or leaky ladies will be okay. And that they can cherish the brilliant bits that come with any darker days.

This doesn't solve the stigma. It would be easy to conclude by chastising myself and all women for not being more upfront, for letting their upset get in the way. But that's dishonest. I *do* know why sometimes I got so upset I couldn't always write, or talk, or joke about it, or I made bad decisions, or nearly drowned: because it *is* rank and depressing and really upsetting. And very (whisper it) very lonely too.

But there must be more. Weaving my way back through the patchwork of my life, as recorded on my electronic devices, I can see evidence – of my body, and the changes in it, the thoughts and the moments and the friends that transformed me, unsettled me and moved me relentlessly along, through my maternal adulthood to my middle years. Browsing my blog, I find myself crying reading about urodynamics and my babies' first words. I am surprised to see how much normal life is in there alongside the incontinence and depression. If I try, I might spot a pattern, not just the full story of how I became *one of those* women, but of how those women could one day move on, pack up their wet pants and become other women too.

I don't want to say 'it' – the whole journey of incontinence – was worth it though. That it taught me to be me, a better me, a wiser woman me. I think it is a sop, an infuriating get-out, when people ask what you have learned from a horrible life event and convince themselves a terrible diagnosis has given you something in some ghastly *quid pro quo*. As if you should be grateful for the opportunity of having every idea you've ever had about yourself and thing you'd like to happen pulverised in public by wicked laughing Fate shoving your hopes and dreams up your big fat arse.

I know I could have been better prepared for some of the things that happened, and wiser, and more well-informed, and definitely more grown-up. But fuck that blame game. Fuck that.

Expecting sick people to rationalise bad luck for us by learning from it isn't helpful or fair. And it really isn't true. There's plenty of life lessons I could have learned from far nicer things happening to me.

So I don't have many answers. But I do have an observation as I sit in the quiet on the eve of another big change. It is an oldie but a goodie. Things do change, and move on, even when you are stuck in the mud and can't see it as it happens. Life's relentlessness means that even the most horrific moments (and trauma, if treated) simply can't last forever. Even the strongest emotions, the worst things like overpowering grief, rage and hate, soften somehow, with time. Even the biggest fears can be addressed. And we all change too.

A decade on, I am a completely different person. I have learned stuff. I have older children now and new worries: not will they ever talk, or write, or put their shoes on the right feet, but will they learn to cross a road, discover happiness, stay healthy, fall in love (oh God), or get sucked into the moral vortex of our crumbling political landscape. I love them as much, maybe more, now they are all arms and legs, have in-jokes without me, and can make their own breakfast.

I am more confident too. And I've learned, most days, to find a way of understanding what has happened to me, placing it in the bigger picture of the world and of my own life. I feel grateful for my luck, and my occasional ability to look for help and good news in what still sometimes feels like a bleak backdrop. I've not learned courage, humility or strength, and I'm not brave for talking about it. I've never been brave, just frustrated, and sad, and cross. And rude. Rude enough to know that it would bolster me up through the worry of talking candidly and honestly about incontinence from a patient's point of view in the hope that someone, anyone, realises she is not alone in finding it difficult and absurd and hilarious and gruesome and dull all at once. Talking sincerely about a stigmatised condition *is* hard, but not talking about it, or feeling all on your own in your soggy state, is even worse.

I want all the leaking people to know that it is okay to feel embarrassed and hopeless or cross. Or to laugh it off or crack brilliant jokes. Or to be shy and private (only laugh it off if it makes you feel better and don't feel the pressure to become a spokesperson if you want to keep it private). But to try, really try, not to let those feelings stop you getting help or finding a way towards improving your condition. I want to say to them all that I know it is hard to explain and even admit the profound shame you might feel. Certainly, it was almost impossible for me. But don't let that beat you down and defeat you. Don't succumb to silence. Reach out.

Yes, I have learned stuff. I now know the flaws of all the characters in Pontypandy when it comes to fire safety, the enchantment of everyday treasures, and the cost of resilience – along with its worth. I understand the power of shame, but also the trick you can play, if the wind is in the right direction, you get the right help, and you face it down and remember it is no more substantial than the Wizard of Oz. Even if shame submerges you, you can always kick back off the bottom towards the light. Especially if you remember this: *Shame is a personal feeling, but here it is caused by other people and the stigma they carry around. It's not yours, it's theirs. Let them have it. Shame that is inflicted on you by prejudice is always unjust. And even if you don't ever want to talk about it, you never have to let it win. Just know you are not alone. And try to be kind to yourself.*

I drain my glass and walk out into the glory of June. 'That one was for you leaky ladies, and men,' I think. 'For all of you, everywhere.'

Epilogue – The Ending: How did I get here?

I don't know when the last time I meet a medical professional in a Urogynaecology department will come. But when I head down there in January 2018, I do not need to catch the professional I meet's name, like I did the first time I met a physio. I know her name. I know more than that. I know about her family, how they've aged, children, grandchildren. I know she thinks about her patients and has a competitive streak a mile wide. She actually does a victory dance when she guesses my size and gets my pessary in, a perfect fit, first go.

She knows about me too – that I like dirty books sometimes myself, though my tastes are more old school than hers, that I love my boys and write about what's happened to me, that I swear too much when I'm nervous. In the next fortnight, she will also learn that I have slightly short fingers compared to the impressive length of my vagina.

Everybody knows that all the best stories need a hook. Or begin with the phrase 'my friend who works in A&E …' You've just had the A&E bit, but this one ends, at least, with an excellent hook, one the size of a knitting needle and a lurid green.

A Saturday, December 2017, large teaching hospital, underground

I am in Carol's office. She is inserting a device I have asked to try, a pessary called a ring with a knob. A ring with a knob. Oh my days!

Vaginal Pessaries

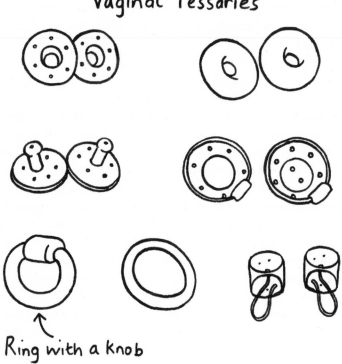

Ring with a knob

The pessary is just one in a long line of things we've tried together, which includes exercises, operations, injections of bulking fluid, waiting to see and more. And it really is called 'a ring with a knob'. Not colloquially, not as a joke by the staff in the unit, as I'd assumed when I first asked about it. But on the packet.

It's a good description; it looks like a plastic donut with a lump or knob on one side. When it is in the right way, that lump gently pushes against your urethra from the other side and holds things like prolapses up, or out of the way, or something. I never do get my anatomy right.

But the pessary is a good thing, because I can manage it myself and unlike pessaries from a long time ago, you can have sex with it in. There are some kinds where you can't. Those are generally used for women who are particularly elderly, unwell and immobile (and who aren't having regular sex). Obviously, some elderly, unwell and immobile women are still sexing away. I hope to become one of them when I hit old age.

Initially, the thought of having such a device felt too much. I was scared I'd forget it and accidentally break my husband's knob, or my ring, or both. But I've been to a conference as a patient representative and spoken to every surgeon, doctor, nurse, GP, physio and researcher I can find there. I think it might give me a new lease of life, some control even, while I think about the rest of my health saga. Another new start, a more continent forties. If I don't like it, I can just use it for special days. High days or holidays. If I want to go out and get drunk and think about medieval poetry, or do Pilates and not wet the mat, or even just go to a supermarket and not worry about the trolley getting too full. Carol and the multidisciplinary team think this is a good option. As long as I'm sensible, and work out how to remove it, I'll be fine.

I believe them. And try to believe her, the confident non-mad Luce who asked for this.

It all seems a bit daunting but once it is in, I stand up. I can feel nothing. Nothing. And I don't leak. I try a shuffle, a step or two. A cough. No, nothing, even though it is the size of a small satsuma.

Carol smiles. 'Go and do some star jumps,' she says. It's an old joke between us. Who would ask an incontinent woman to do that?

I get out of the hospital having not pissed at all on the stairs, even though I'm using a walking stick so expecting pain to make things harder. She's asked me to walk around for half an hour, try it out. As it's nearly Christmas, I decide to buy her a present. I find an orchid that looks a bit like a fanny. Also, it is high maintenance and unique. Like me. I've met more than one woman in my 40 years who has called their bits their flower, so it feels right.

I take it back with some treats for everyone in Urodynamics. I forgive them. Carol is embarrassed, and pleased, I think, but surprised. It's weird, us being opposites, even if it's just for a second: me confident and hopeful, her slightly taken aback.

'You don't have to do that,' she says. Proud and true.

'I wanted to,' I say. Feeling like nothing will be right or enough. 'You've given me a lot.' I don't know how to explain it to her: every time they did something for me, made me a new woman, helped me out, I wanted to buy gifts, to say thank you properly, do *something*, but I was almost always too upset. Or shocked. Or ill. Or ashamed. And it felt too weird coming down here without an appointment. I only did it once to leave a scarf for Lizzie the physio after my last ever session with her. I had to scuttle away. It felt wrong, intrusive.

But maybe that's okay, to start to want to move on.

She shows me how to take the thing out. It looks easy. I don't find it easy at all. I can barely manage to get a hold of it up my own bits. It's awful, grasping around up there.

She turns her back on me.

'There's nothing worse than somebody watching you while you're pawing your own Minnie,' says Carol to explain, sighing to herself as she stares at the sink. 'Nothing.'

'I don't know,' I say. 'Those urodynamic tests have to be up there.'

But even if nobody's looking, I still can't reach the ring of silicon stuck up my snatch. I can't grab it, let alone pull it out. I can't imagine the angle it is at. Or with what force it will fly into orbit if I ever get my fingers on it.

I try not to grunt. But my fingers are too stubby for my own vagina. I fail.

We discuss options. She thinks when I can relax at home, I'll probably be able to remove it if necessary, and I can always come in and get them to do it, if for any reason it needs to come out sooner and I can't manage. It's Christmas. I'm soaked in goodwill and optimism. And despite my ham-fisted attempts at dislodging it, it is still in the right place. It's a sign. We decide to see how it works anyway ...

It was the night before Christmas when I felt something like a flip. A movement at first, then the irritating and difficult sensation of the pessary hard inside me and pressing upwards. It feels like the knob has moved right round. To be fair to it, to the poor silicon ring, the rest of my body has read a different script. Incontinence be damned, my body now has arthritis to think about. I'm 40 but it clearly enjoys the ride when it comes to premature diseases of ageing.

I can feel the pessary now for sure. It is a bit like having a sweep as it touches my cervix. I think, 'Houston, we have a problem.'

After a four-hour session, including two baths and some googling, I finally remove it. Young women all over the world, blogging and posting on YouTube about how their vaginas work and how to fit a menstrual cup, save me. Women embracing their own physiology and experience rather than being cowed by the stigma that surrounds it. This is *Our Bodies, Ourselves* for the digital age. They show me theirs; I get to know mine.

I think, 'Merry Christmas to all, and to all a good night.' And thank the Lord for this new generation who have finally stopped giving a shit.

I clean my pessary and put it in the cupboard, then tuck a roll of Sellotape in my bra. I have Christmas to embrace and stockings to fill. I'll try it again on Boxing Day ...

We head back to Carol's Saturday clinic. We tried again, it has flipped again – but I kept a diary. It isn't the thing, which works really well; it is my other health issues creeping in. But I'm struck by insecurity and self-blame anyway and fixate on it being the fault of my design.

'Is the shape a problem? Is the ridge at the start of my vagina too high?' I squeak.

'I think that one's just the way you're made,' says Carol, reassuringly.

'But is it too long and too baggy, is this why I've had all these issues?' I ask of my own foof.

Carol stares. Ten years of incontinence and I'm still a buffoon with no body knowledge, even now I've embraced my inner and outer fem.

'You are very small down there.'

I look at her.

'It's TIGHT, Lady. Long, but tight. That's why you can't reach it,' says Carol.

'Oh,' I say, mollified and slightly proud. 'Surely not.'

'You deserve that one,' she adds. I decide to take it where I can get it.

Doesn't solve the problem though. Carol can get it out, with her fingers. And zip it in, superfast, leaving it snuggly in the right place. I can get it in, though only by posting it with a manoeuvre Carol calls 'like a penny in a slot'. But I can't retrieve it. And I'll never be able to think 'in for a penny' again.

'I always worry I'm getting the answers wrong, you know? That I've let you all down being back here,' I say, to explain my faltering. 'And now I can't even get it out. I am the worst patient.'

'No,' she says, kindly as ever. 'No. It's just we just don't like to see people having to come back. We just wish you didn't have to be here.'

She tells me it will always be retrievable. I worry other professionals might fumble if they aren't used to pessaries and she offers to show me the 'crochet hook', her nickname for a medical instrument specifically designed to retrieve rogue devices, as it would be the sort of thing someone might use if needed. She brings it in. Green and enormous, it looks like it is used for backstreet abortions. It has a special packet.

'It's sterile,' Carol explains.

'I should bloody well hope so,' I think.

My fem rage activates, as does my fear. I am about to wobble but then it hits. Optimism. In a wave just as hard and deathly strong as depression ever was.

It's too dangerous for patients to keep a hook at home and use it on themselves. I'm not surprised: it's massive. I don't sink though. I feel like running away when I see it, but I go steady instead and think 'no guts, no glory'.

Knowing the hook is there calms me down and I take a picture so that if I ever need to I can show someone medical the implement that will get the pessary out, and she assures me it won't come to that – they will fit me into clinic if it ever gets stuck again. I won't give up, I will make this work. Or make the next thing work.

Carol opens the appointment files on the hospital PC.

'And you know we'll have to think about the future,' she says.

I feel a bit emotional and blurt out that I have written a book. About incontinence and leaking and women and emotion. I explain that I've melded together her and her partners in crime, the other brilliant nurse specialists, and I've named them Carol, who I love.

'I like that,' she says.

'I didn't want to embarrass you, but I didn't want you to think I didn't know who you were,' I explain. I tell her about John Skelton, and how I've pieced it all together. And then I whisper it. That I know it isn't quite a goodbye.

'I'll always be like this, won't I? Or at least, I'm always going to be someone with issues, at risk of it getting worse again, especially as I get older, aren't I, Carol? I'm 40 now. I'm going to have to work at it. Especially with the menopause. Is that right?'

'Ach,' Carol sighs to herself. 'Ach,' in the way only Scottish people can, even if they don't say it often. She has the kindness and respect to turn round to look at me, and hold me with her steady, honest gaze.

'Ach, love. You'll always have to keep an eye on it. It will be something there in you.'

'Will I be back then?' I ask.

'Maybe,' she says. She's wary of false promises, good or bad. But not afraid of truth. She looks at me again. 'We'll keep in touch. We'll see what happens. If you have to speak to the surgery boys again …?'

'It's okay,' I say. My voice is only a bit small. 'I like the Waz Wizard, and his children.'

'That's what you call them?' She laughs.

We have reached an understanding. There's lots of things that could happen. New techniques. New ideas. Who knows what my forties, fifties, sixties, seventies will hold?

'You can do it,' she adds.

I give her a kiss on the cheek, a firm nod, and a saucy wink for all the dirty books and fanny talk and kindness we've had to endure and embrace. And then I walk out. The patient toilet is open, but I don't need to cry in there again. There are women in the waiting room. Carol hums and walks to the reception desk.

'I love Saturday clinic,' she says to herself, but also to all of us. 'It's the familiar faces.' Being part of this club is not so bad after all.

And then I feel it. A smile. I'm not grinning, obviously. I'm not *happy* that my initial assessment all those years ago, that I was a forever broken leaky lady, was fairly close to the mark. That incontinence will always be just around the corner, if I'm lucky, in another room, but waiting, like depression, to pounce again.

I smile nonetheless. This is not the end. I can't feel it as the end anymore. The honesty helps. The acceptance, validation, that I will be carrying on and being mindful of myself, rather than cured, that this is part of a longer story even, is okay. Rather than being terrified or angry, I feel free. Weird, yes. But mostly free.

I don't feel like I'm being fired or abandoned. Just that although coming back somewhere for help is as certain as death and taxes and never losing the last 4lb of baby weight, it doesn't have to be straight away and I've got this. I know how I got here.

My situation is stoutly, proudly, solidly exactly what it is. And I'm okay with it. With the probably, maybe, definitely, defiantly coming back being on the cards. And with who and what *I* am: someone whose incontinence wasn't ideal but who has plans in place and hopes, and I can wrestle it under control and stop it defining me. I'm good, with holding what I have for now and knowing maybe more will be needed sometime in the future. The final sign-off session with a women's health specialist might never come.

I'm caught by the spirit of something, Christmas Present? Christmas Future? Hogmanay? Certainly, something catches in my throat. My pessary is in. I won't wee even if I cry. I let a tear prick the corner of my eye and wave to Carol, as she walks back up the corridor with her next patient to start again at mending things. I smile at the receptionist and pencil in a phone call for next season. In the strip lighting, I'm laid bare, but I'm walking. And I'm not frightened anymore.

What if you are leaky too?

A short-term incontinence survival guide

Ten things I learned the hard way, so you don't have to.

1. Do your bloody pelvic floor exercises

Yes, they're boring. Yes, you've probably got something better to do. Yes, you're busy. Yes, checking if you are doing them right can be a bit like wanking. And yes, at home you can't actually see any improvements like you can with other sorts of physio, which might feel disheartening. But pelvic floor exercises (aka Kegels) work for almost everyone to some degree and there are many places online where you can find out how to do them right even if you aren't ready or able to go to a clinic. Usually they don't take that long to work either. Just six sessions with a physio, or even a few weeks on your own, might be all you need to get dry. But do them, properly, with help if you need it, to make sure you are exercising the right bits, and then remember to keep at it so you can get dry as a desert and stay that way. Don't cheat by only doing the short-burst holds because they are quick and easy. We've all been there, but the long ones help too.

2. Be sensible.

E.g though wearing pads 'just in case' isn't ideal, if you need them for a bit, use them. Find the ones that work for you (you might need to experiment a bit) and then bingo, a stop gap while you work out how you can get help. But get help where you can: download the Squeezy app or similar, look it all up online, speak to your doctor, a physio, your yoga/fitness/Pilates instructor. Many people are able to see incontinence for the shitshow it really is and can talk to you about it and support you.

Also – DON'T STOP DRINKING WATER TO AVOID LEAKING. It doesn't work or help and comes with other risks, e.g dehydration.

3. Embrace the uniform as a stop gap if you have to

It's boring, but it is slightly better than walking home soaking. I went for indiscernible clothes changes, preferably one colour, that skimmed over both the baby belly leftovers and the bulging pad-filled knicker area. Ideally, I'd also pick things that folded small and didn't need ironing, because I'm lazy and wanted to be able to put them in a changing bag.

I became a huge fan of the slouch bag and sensible large pants with black leggings, dresses and long cardigans. Triple protection. You will find your own solution.

4. Incontinence and sex is the biggest taboo for a reason

It may be unmentionable but sexual dysfunction as a result of incontinence is not uncommon; medical research suggests between 25 and 50 per cent of women with urinary incontinence experience it. Which is difficult, depressing and horrible. Just horrible. So, it doesn't make you weird if talking about the problem or having sex or thinking about sex is hard to handle. But look at those stats: between a quarter and a half of leaky ladies have some kind of 'in the bedroom' issue so please don't let a sense that you are weird, or broken, or fussy, or disgusting put you off asking for help, or let it keep you from talking to your partner if you possibly can. I know that's hard. It is another lonely road for anyone incontinent, but I hope you feel bolstered by knowing that once again you aren't alone. And also that there is potential for you to get much, much better. This does not automatically mean the end of your sexual life.

On a practical note, if you find sex brings out the worst in your leaking, or are worrying about it before you've tried it, then your first stop should be finding a protection for your mattress that works for you so you feel comfortable and safe all night. There are proper products available for this, or you could go for borrowing the water-proof sheet from the cot or crib once your baby is over it if it isn't too noisy. (Or try using the disposable maternity bed pads used in hospitals, which you can buy from chemists, and use fairly discreetly.)

Also, when I first became incontinent, night times were difficult even if there was no dirty deed. I didn't wet the bed in a traditional sense, though some people do. I was accidently wetting my pants while I was in bed, catching my bedding in the crossfire. But sorting out some coverage and sheeting is essential to feeling less overwhelmed by laundry and the drudge of it all and making it less likely you'll have to shell out for a new mattress.

5. The world doesn't stop in sympathy for trauma or personal disasters

It's brutal but true. You'll still get allergies, hay fever, colds and chest infections, and sad things will happen that make you bawl, even though the universe should give you a break. And life goes on. It is shocking at first but that's why support for continence issues, birth trauma and depression is so important wherever you find it. I've put lots of links at the back that might be helpful.

6. Tests will be okay – especially if you take someone with you

There's so much to write about the exquisite horror, hilarity, absurdity and grimness of tests focused on your privates, though they are always better if you are wearing lucky socks and have someone waiting for you afterwards if that's at all possible.

Mostly though, they are fine, even the rank ones. People are nice, and professionals know it sucks to be the one whose bits are on display – even if they sometimes forget and get over-excited by your particularly great injury or can't hide their boredom that you are their tenth fanny in a row.

Take an MRI. They are fine but can feel a bit loud and stressful as they happen. It is a bit like being Sandra Bullock in *Gravity*, getting drunk on space vodka but without George Clooney to hold your hand. Pretty much everyone who has an MRI finds it weird. Remember, it's in nobody's interest for you to panic, or for you to not have a test you need, so you can be honest with the nurses/technicians, and/or the doctor who ordered it, and ask for them to help explain what's going on. Also, as with any toilet tests, don't feel bad about just wanting a cup of tea and to let the world go fuck itself for a bit afterwards.

So, go. And remember, this is a book with comedy in it, where I focused on the grim side, but I still went along and so can you. And *obviously* you don't have to make it into a stand-up routine – you can approach tests in your own way.

7. Don't call them nappies if it breaks your heart

If your incontinence is really bad, you may have to do away with knickers and use disposable pants. The Americans call these adult diapers, some call them nappies; I found avoiding that vocab made me feel less wretched.

Outrageously, they are expensive. And horrible. When I first needed them, they were only flowery white ones. The flowers were so insulting, as if the flourish of prettiness masks the utilitarian sizing and general gloom. They've improved a bit now and they are fairly comfortable. You can also get washable ones, and some – finally – in black, so you don't get the white-crotch glow.

As I said before, for some people it feels heartbreaking to buy them, but doing it the first time teaches you the most important lesson of all: *Incontinence requires pragmatism, even when it feels like it will kill you. And pragmatism? You can do that.*

On that note, I can't include financial advice, but I regret not acting on impulse 10 years ago and investing my pension in incontinence products. As we all age, the leaky bum boom times are coming. It's just a thought.

8. Explore your options

I don't advocate having surgery, not having surgery, or any specific exercise or regime or tools or devices for you to use. I've never seen your fanny or a jug of your piss. That's what medical professionals, experienced healthcare workers, pelvic health specialists and their support staff are for – to impart their specific knowledge to specific patients with all their expertise. And you can ask questions, ask for second opinions, ask advice. Write it down, take a friend, type some words on your phone and hand it over – people working with difficult conditions know they are hard to talk about.

I do advocate finding a way to feel you are finding your way with purpose though. It's also worth restating that the mesh operation was never on the table for me, as a first option, given my specific case. And even the second time I needed some help to navigate and digest the research. But with that case in partic- ular in mind, carefully considering the research and risks, with a doctor who can talk it through with you properly, is key.

9. Don't let the stigma control you – connections with others can kill it

Stigma is awful, as is shame. It isn't fair and it contributes to terrible things like depression, self-loathing and crying in toilets, as well as larger social problems like incontinence not getting the funding it deserves and incontinent people still suffering disproportionately, despite there being hundreds of millions of us around the globe.

That doesn't mean you will wake up tomorrow able to face- down thousands of years of oppression, jokes and skewed language that belittles you and makes you feel disgusting. Or, sadly, that you can force other people to be enlightened about talking about stuff that makes them uncomfortable. And you don't have to air your dirty knickers in public like I did. There's no pressure. Just remember, stigma isn't the boss of you. You are.

You don't have to talk about it, but there are places you can if you want to, especially if you are feeling isolated and rotten or you are also starting to feel depressed. There are lots of places to go and opportunities for care, from talking things through to medications, support groups to charities specialising in birth trauma, and continence and related emotional issues. You really should get help – see the back of this book for a start.

The Internet has transformed the embarrassed patient's experience, with forums full of people who have the same things going on, but you can also just remind yourself of the numbers – there are other people like you everywhere, and twitter hashtags you can join in or lurk around if you don't want to reach out. There are lots of ways of sharing experience – reading about other people can be just as helpful as talking if you aren't up for going public. Please remember though, anyone can *sound* like an expert, it is always wise to check anything you are unsure about with a qualified medical professional.

Remember too, no body is perfect but all bodies deserve care. People know bodies break down. Mostly they are just sad for you (or thinking about their own inadequacies far too much to focus on yours).

Also, if the stigma doesn't bother you, that's fine too. Some of the experts I spoke to felt women were so sure that they should be ashamed that they didn't feel like they could say things like, 'I don't really want surgery, thanks, I'd rather try a pessary and occasional pads if that's okay.' You can do that, there's no one forcing you to do anything you don't want to do with your leaky bits.

10. This isn't your fault
It isn't. You don't deserve it, it isn't fair, and it is absolutely dire to have to cope with a taboo medical problem. At some point you will probably need to take a deep breath and draw on reserves

that you don't really think you have. Which isn't fair either. So if you need a minute to stomp a bit because it isn't fair, here it is. It sucks, and I'm sorry. Not pitying, just sorry.

If depression is creeping up on you too, you can also feel rightly indignant and destroyed by the cruel BOGOF of incontinence and depression. That can literally BOG OFF though; it is rubbish, you haven't failed at being brave or resourceful enough, there is evidence which shows just how crushing incontinence is for lots and lots and lots of us. You've just had bad luck.

So, go steady. Feel sad and lost if you need to, but at some point, when you get a second to yourself to galvanise some strength, you are going to find some help, the sort that works for you – and the tools to keep yourself going. From pads to physio, physicians to a jumper round your waist, surgery to advocacy, counselling to jokes with your friends.

Though word to the wise: trauma, depression, anxiety, panic attacks, thinking you can't go on – these are all real conditions, which need real help. You can't dust those aside and hope looking on the bright side will easily sort them, which is why I've added extra mind help links at the back of this book too.

Remember: it *isn't* selfish to want help, or silly. You aren't making a fuss. You *are allowed* to want to be clean and better and not depressed. And you might well be someone for whom conservative (or non-surgical) measures work wonders – you could be someone who is easily cured. Nobody *has* to sit around in pissy knickers, not having all the fun and exercise and sex, especially women who have been told to 'shh' about it all their entire lives. There's no need to put up with anything that makes you feel awful, affects your sex life and relationships, causes other health problems, and puts you at a social disadvantage. The silence is oppressive but we're starting to shout over it.

I know that's easy for me to say. But I also know you can get this sorted. I promise.

And one for luck: *throw away your best knickers if they are haunting you*
I tortured myself with my knicker drawer from 'before', bulging with colourful lacy numbers that once made me feel good. I figure there are four choices.

1   Keep them if you find them motivating for doing your exercises and improving what can be improved.
2   Keep them, but tidied away, if you can treat them as a memento from a different time.
3   Wear them and be damned, if you won't be heartbroken by soiling them – who says people who wet themselves occasionally can't piss on posh pants? Not me.
4   Chuck them out. For God's sake, if you are the sort of person who finds them an everyday reminder of what you once were and life's unfairness then get rid! If you can afford it, chuck the lot. Ideally you need to wear more comfy ones that work with pads. Get yourself some nice ones when you are feeling and doing better. (You can always get some fuck-me lipstick or whatever else tickles your feel-good fancy in the meantime.)

Talking to doctors about your private parts – written with GP Rachel Boyce

This book isn't a self-help guide and I have no medical training. If you are having trouble with incontinence or depression, the good news is that however hard it might feel, there are absolutely loads of places you can go to get easy help and good advice. LOADS.

For incontinence, the most obvious first port of call is your GP, who will know exactly what services are available to you. If you find it hard to know what to say to them, there are plenty of approaches.

All GPs have postgraduate training in women's health and continence, but your practice may well have a GP who specialises in it. Take a look at the practice website before you book, or ask reception whether they have any GPs with a special interest.

It is also completely okay to prefer to see a female or male GP if you think that will help you feel more comfortable, or to ask for a chaperone (another trained adult, often reception or other surgery staff) to come in with you. Receptionists are very used to this request, as are the clinicians. In fact, it's quite a handy thing if you can't bear to tell the receptionist exactly what the issue is: 'Could I see a female doctor please, as it's a personal problem [about my pelvic floor?]' Receptionists read between the lines and will often steer such a request towards the correct person.

How you talk about what's happening to you will always be very personal. I went for a bald statement, and occasionally choice language, but you are likely far more polite. The key is this: you aren't the only person going through this and most medical professionals will understand if you are embarrassed (even if they tell you not to be). Doctors know not everyone walks around using words like urethra or bladder or bowels or prolapse and they're very likely to know exactly what you mean if you say you are leaking, wetting yourself, or having accidents, and to know how to ask the right questions to work out exactly what is going wrong and what help you need.

Remember, most doctors are doctors because they find the human body totally fascinating rather than disgusting. All doctors, in their time, have been covered in all bodily fluids (not just blood, snot, poo and wee, but really obscure stuff like pus and amniotic fluid) and they really don't feel the disgust that patients often do about bodies.

Also, it makes not the slightest bit of difference whether a patient has shaved their legs or their bits. It makes no difference at all to how easy or hard the examination is and what the findings are. None. So try not to worry on those scores.

Working with a GP I know, we've come up with a list of statements that you could take in with you if you are reading a hard copy of this book, or show on your tablet if you are reading by ebook.

They aren't completely exhaustive, but they highlight the most common symptoms and should also get you started even if they only apply in part to you.

Your GP will have heard and seen a great deal in their working life. You won't shock them and they will probably be pleased to see a patient who can be helped; incontinence can often be easily sorted with straightforward and non-surgical measures like doing the exercises yourself at home, minor tweaks to how much you drink and when, or how often you go to the loo, and finding the right sort of exercise.

A word on GP receptionists. These members of staff are often criticised for asking personal questions, though this is not out of nosiness and is part of their job. It is just because they are helping GPs to work out who needs seeing when. If they ask for a summary of why you want an appointment, you could use one of the more general phrases from the start of the list below.

What should you say?

Writing this book taught me that a great many women, and men, however confident and outgoing they are, find incontinence very hard to talk about. Here are some things to get the conversation started and some short sentences you could say to highlight some of the most common specific issues.

Conversation starters

- I am having trouble with my pelvic floor;
- I'd like to talk to you about some problems I am having when I go to the toilet;
- I am worried about my leaking wee/urine and/or from my bottom/back passage;
- I think I need some help with incontinence/leaking.

Specific issues you might want to highlight – the phrases work for poo/faeces/stools as well as wee/urine …

- It is painful when I wee;
- My wee is cloudy/there is blood in it;
- I need to go to the toilet a lot;
- I am leaking wee/urine when I cough/run/jump/ sneeze, etc;
- I am having trouble with controlling my pelvic floor/ I can't hold wee/urine in like I used to be able to;
- I need to get up in the night several times to go to the toilet;

- I find I suddenly need to go to the toilet when I am not expecting it;
- I sometimes leak wee/urine for no reason;
- I leak wee/urine when I am upset or emotional;
- There has been a big change in how much and how often I wee/urinate;
- Sometimes when I am going to the toilet, I carry on weeing or urinating when I think I have finished;
- I am leaking wee/urine during sex;
- I am wetting the bed;
- I can't wee when I feel the urge;
- When I need the toilet urgently, it is hard for me to move quickly and I am scared I will fall;
- I can't feel it when I wee;
- I am having trouble with incontinence and it is making me anxious or depressed;

Or just write down what the issue is on a piece of paper/your phone and take it with you and show the doctor.

What will happen when you go to the GP?

Your GP will ask you how it's affecting your life, and this is your chance to talk through options you might like to explore, what you're worried about and what you're expecting to happen (for example, if you're hoping to be referred to a physiotherapist or to use a pessary).

They may also ask questions about:

- Any complications you had in pregnancy or labour if you have had children;
- Your bowel habits;
- Your drinking or diet;
- Any underlying illnesses or health conditions you may have, or previous surgeries;

- Any medication you are taking;
- Contraception and maybe if it's affecting your sex life.

You may need to give a sample of urine. Your GP or receptionist will ask you to do this using a special plastic container. If you want to be really helpful, bring a sample along to your appointment or do one in the surgery loos before you sit down to wait your turn – receptionists will hand you an empty urine sample pot for bringing to an appointment if you ask them (for free), and you can even buy the sample pots from pharmacies if you prefer.

Don't bring it in any old container though, it needs to be sterile. Ideally, doctors want the bit from the mid-stream, i.e. just after you start weeing, but really any sample (in the correct container) is better than none.

Some GPs have a jug in the toilet at the surgery which you can rinse out, wee into, and then pour the wee into the container. In others they might have disposable cups from which you can fill, then tip the sample into the white- or red-topped bottle before it goes to the lab.

If you are asked to collect a stool sample it is likely you will be given a special pot which may also have a small spatula-like tool to use to scoop up a small amount of the poo. It is important that you catch your sample in the pot or on some loo roll before you scoop some off, because it mustn't fall into the toilet water which will contaminate the sample. It sounds hard but if you can reach to wipe your bottom yourself you should be okay.

Some people prefer to poo directly into a clean container that they can throw away afterwards, and then just use the spatula to get the sample into the pot. It is important to keep the inside of the pot and the spatula sterile, so don't let them touch anything apart from the poo. If you have diarrhoea then wrap tissue/toilet paper around the outside of the pot to catch the spills and catch the watery motion in the pot. Remember to wash your hands when you are finished.

Being examined by a doctor

It's sometimes hard for a GP to have enough time to take a good history and examine a patient in one appointment, so they may ask you to come back to be examined in a separate appointment.

An examination would usually involve something called a 'bimanual': the doctor puts two gloved fingers inside your vagina and the other hand on your lower abdomen. They may ask you to cough a little to see if they can feel a prolapse or bulge. Then they might want to do a speculum examination (the same type of examination that you have when you have a smear test). This uses a clear plastic disposable speculum that looks a bit like a duck's beak to see whether the walls of the vagina are lax or damaged in any way.

If you have male body parts you may need an examination to check whether your prostate gland is enlarged. Your prostate is normally around the size of a walnut and lives under the bladder. It is normal for them to get bigger with age, but it is important to be vigilant as an enlarged prostate can be a sign of some serious problems. Changes there can cause symptoms which range from the irritating to the alarming. Such as slowing down or stopping the flow of your wee, making it dribble, or making you need to pass urine more often (and at night). It could even make your wee contain blood too or be linked to erectile dysfunction. If you are getting help for those sorts of symptoms, your examination is likely to include a manual check of your prostate, in which your doctor will use a gloved finger and insert it into your bottom. It sounds daunting but is very quick and effective as it allows the doctor to check for any changes in size. Your doctor may also ask you to have a blood test.

If you are referred to a hospital or physiotherapy setting, it is possible you will need to be examined again or have to give additional samples or have some imaging or other tests. This is so they can make sure they organise the most appropriate help and treatment for you. Hang on in there, as Carol used to say, you can do it.

Getting help and information
for a broken body

There is a wealth of information available online, from chat services and helplines with physiotherapists and other experts to chat rooms, which can offer some comfort, solace in speaking to other wet-knicker-warriors and continence patients and survivors, and support in times of trouble. However, before you start any self-care, it is always a good idea to have your bits checked out so that you have a clear idea what exactly your problem is. There are many types of incontinence and sometimes people have more than one at the same time. It is definitely a good idea to find out what you are dealing with before you make major changes.

Belows are some websites I found particularly useful. Some use different approaches, some are related to famous brands, but I don't endorse any one in particular and I have not been paid to promote any of them.

- www.pelvicroar.org – Campaigners working to improve information and evidence-based care, and to raise awareness about continence and other gynaecological issues;
- www.continenceproductadvisor.org – The Continence Product Advisor website is a not-for-profit venture and includes information about the different kinds of products available, allowing you to look at what might work for you, and search according to type of incontinence and any other issues you might specifically

want to bear in mind – for example, mobility, how well you can see. It is a collaboration between the International Consultation on Incontinence (ICI) and the International Continence Society (ICS);

- www.ics.org – International Continence Society. Industry body with stats, research and fact sheets;
- www.nhs.uk/Livewell/incontinence/Pages/ Gettinghelp.aspx – Brilliant clear information from the UK's National Health Service, including videos on continence and what help is available;
- www.gussetgrippers.co.uk – Excellent resources from physiotherapist turned stand-up Elaine, who is saving the world one fanjo at a time, starting with a website designed to answer lots of difficult questions people have but are often too afraid to ask;
- www.bladderandboweluk.co.uk – An excellent charity with a wealth of straight-talking, easy-to-understand and helpful resources, stories from others with a variety of conditions and a free helpline;
- www.tena.co.uk/women/ – Advice and resources for women from pad manufacturers, with the option to buy their products direct if you can't face the supermarket aisle of shame or if you are unable to leave the house easily and would find delivery helped that;
- www.tena.co.uk/men/ – As above, for men and male continence products;
- www.alwaysdiscreet.co.uk/en-gb – Website and product information from Always about their Discreet ranges, including pants and pads. Again, information, people's real experiences, videos and information about leaking;
- www.kegel8.co.uk – Website for electronic pelvic floor exercising devices, which also contains a wealth of information and an informative blog with a whole host of embarrassing and upsetting issues discussed frankly

and clearly. Set up by a remarkable woman who put her own experiences to excellent use helping develop tools for others;

- www.squeezyapp.com – Recommended by NHS app library, info on finding a physiotherapist and pelvic floor exercises;
- www.eric.org.uk – Children's bowel and bladder charity with wealth of information;
- www.freedomfromfistula.org.uk – Charitable work curing fistula and working with birth-injured mothers in the community;
- www.marslord.co.uk – Maternal care information and commentary, and the introduction to the role of doulas;
- www.csp.org.uk – Chartered Society of Physiotherapists. Info including Personal Training Your Pelvic Floor leaflet;
- www.incontinence.co.uk – News, studies, info on incontinence for men and women;
- www.pelvicfloorfirst.org.au – Australian government funded site with evidence-based resources and videos and advice.

If you are having trouble relating to a difficult or traumatic birth, or birth injuries, specific advice is available from charities including the Birth Trauma Association (www.birthtraumaassociation.org.uk) and The MASIC Foundation (who specialise in help and policy relating to those with anal sphincter injuries in childbirth: www.masic.org.uk).

Getting help and information for a broken mind

Remember, your brain is just another part of your body, which also deserves care and attention

I have written a great deal about the effects on my mind of a traumatic birth and difficult physical condition. Like incontinence, it can feel very, very hard to go and ask for help or explain how you are feeling. You can feel lonely, frustrated, tearful, isolated, sad, exhausted, desperate. However, also like incontinence, there is a great deal that can be done, from medication to other therapies, through the NHS and privately.

Your GP, midwife or health visitor is an excellent place to start to find out what help you can get and how to start working towards recovery.

Online help
As with incontinence, there is no substitute for speaking to a trained medical professional. However, there are several services available online and by phone, especially if you need to speak to someone urgently because you are feeling really low or bad. I found some of the following sources very helpful or had them recommended to me:

- www.samaritans.org – The Samaritans offer a wealth of services to listen to you if you are feeling really down, or even suicidal. They are extremely helpful, kind and experienced and can make a real difference, even if you feel that no one could possibly help or understand. You

can email jo@samaritans.org or ring 116 123 (UK) or
116 123 (ROI). You can also visit your local Samaritans
branch (easy to Google or find on their site) or write to
them at: Freepost RSRB-KKBY-CYJK, PO Box 9090,
STIRLING, FK8 2SA. They are open 24 hours a day,
365 days a year. If you need them *right now*, it is best to
ring. The call is FREE. You don't have to be suicidal to
call them;

- www.nhs.uk/livewell/mentalhealth/Pages/
  Mentalhealthhome.aspx – Lots of information about
  mental health, and how you can access the right services
  for you. The website is easy to access. You could also
  call your GP or NHS 111;
- www.mind.org.uk – Excellent specialist mental health
  charity, who were also very helpful;
- www.rcpsych.ac.uk/mental-health/problems-
  disorders/post-natal-depression – Site from Royal
  College of Psychiatrists with clear information about
  PND and other maternal mental health conditions;
- #pndhour – A Twitter hashtag for weekly community
  voices and experience. PND and related issues;
- www.slingthemesh.wordpress.com – Campaigning and
  support for mesh-injured patients;
- Private Facebook group, Mashed up by Mesh –
  A specific support forum for those feeling suicidal
  following mesh surgery;
- www.mentalhealth-uk.org/help-and-information/
  conditions/depression/more-information/ – Support
  for people affected by mental health problems, including their friends, family and carers, with useful links to
  mental health charities and resources;
- www.pandasfoundation.org.uk/ – Information, support
  and advice for parents and their networks who need
  support with perinatal mental illness.

References

Opening quotes

- 'stigma – a mark of disgrace associated with a particular circumstance, quality, or person': *Oxford Living Dictionaries*, www. en.oxforddictionaries.com;
- 'Bladder weakness alone affects 1 in 3 people and is more common than hay fever': Campaign pack for World Continence Week 2019, www.wfip.org/world-continence-week-2019.

Introduction

- 'One in three women wet themselves, and about one in 10 have problems controlling their bowels' https://www.ics.org/ Publications/ICI_5/INCONTINENCE.pdf
- Craig P, Dieppe P, Macintyre S, Michie SN, I., Petticrew M. *Developing and evaluating complex interventions*: the new Medical Research Council guidance. MMJ. 2008;337(a1655).
- Hunskaar S., Lose G., Sykes D., Voss S, *The prevalence of urinary incontinence in women in four European countries*. BJUI. 2004(93):324–30.
- Woodley S.J., Boyle R., Cody J.D., Mørkved S, E.C. H-S. *How effective are pelvic floor muscle exercises undertaken during pregnancy or after birth for preventing or treating incontinence?* Cochrane Library, 2017.
- Schreiber Pedersen L., Lose G., Høybye M.T., Elsner S., Waldmann A., M. R. *Prevalence of urinary incontinence among women and analysis of potential risk factors in Germany and Denmark*. Acta Obstet Gynecol Scand. 2017;98(8):939–48.
- Lang K., Alexander I.M., Simon J., Sussman M., Lin I., Menzin J., et al. *The impact of multimorbidity on quality of life among midlife women: findings from a U.S. nationally*

representative survey. Journal of Women's Health. 2015;24(5):374–83.

- 'empowered with the skills, confidence and knowledge needed to play an active role in making informed decisions about their own health care and management of their chronic condition': www.bmj.com/rapid-response/2011/10/29/research-expert-patient-concept.

Chapter 1: Speaking up

- 'In 2016, 38 per cent of UK women with incontinence issues were too embarrassed to tell a health professional about it at all': www.nct.org.uk/about-us/news-and-views/news/breaking-taboo-incontinence-after-childbirth;
- 'Kegels (first published descriptions, 1948)': Kegel, Arnold H.: *The Nonsurgical Treatment of Genital Relaxation*, West, Med & Surg. 31: 213–216, May, 1948; Kegel, Arnold H.: *Progressive Resistance Exercise to the Functional Restoration of the Perineal Muscles*, Am. J. Obst. & Gynec. 56: 238–248, August, 1948; Kegel, Arnold H.: *The Physiologic Treatment of Poor Tone and Function of the Genital Muscles and of Urinary Stress Incontinence*, West, J. Surg., Obst. & Gynec. 57: 527–535, November, 1949.

Chapter 2: Childbirth expectations

- 'There are studies on how the traumatic nature of TV and film births contributes to birth fear amongst expectant mothers.' https://rdcu.be/b2nVV
- 'Is it realistic?' the portrayal of pregnancy and childbirth in the media Ann Luce, Marilyn Cash, Vanora Hundley, Helen Cheyne, Edwin van Teijlingen and Catherine Angell.

Chapter 3: Childbirth reality

- *'My mother groan'd! my father wept. / Into the dangerous world I leapt'*: 'Infant Sorrow', William Blake, *Songs of Experience*, (1794). *The Poems of William Blake, A New Edition*, (Shepherd), Pickering and Chatto (1887);

Chapter 5: Six-week check

- 'Sylvia's clear that love set him going "like a fat gold watch"': from "Morning Song" from Ariel by Sylvia Plath, Faber & Faber (1965). Copyright © 1961 by Ted Hughes. Used by permission of HarperCollins Publishers.

Chapter 7: Depression

- 'Women with incontinence are, in fact, almost twice as likely to develop PND': McMaster University, 'Urinary incontinence doubles risk of postpartum depression', ScienceDaily, 20 June 2011: www.sciencedaily.com/releases/2011/06/110620103941.htm;
- "'Only connect! That was the whole of her sermon …'": quoted with kind permission of The Provost and Scholars of King's College, Cambridge and The Society of Authors as the E.M. Forster Estate.

Chapter 8: Survival

- Bristol Stool Chart: Based on Rome Foundation's original BSFS copyright 2016 Rome Foundation, Inc. All Rights Reserved;
- 'part of the sign-off criteria post-birth': This article arrives much later, but typifies the comparisons I was hearing even at the time: www.theguardian.com/commentisfree/2016/nov/02/french-mothers-bladder-incontinence-nadia-sawalha
- 'key in lock syndrome': www.obgyn.net/hysterectomy/urinary-incontinence-closet-condition, *Urinary Incontinence: A Closet Condition!* Mark Smith, Jr, MD 7 October 2011.

Chapter 9: Booze

- "'she's got a face like a pig's ear 'brystled' with hair'": *The Tunning of Eleanour Rumming* from *The Poetical Works of John Skelton, Volume 1*, principally according to the edition of Revd. Alexander Dyce, *In Three Volumes. Volume 1*, Riverside, Cambridge, 1855, p.110. Modern translations my own;
- "*Then began she to wepe, And forthwith fell on slepe. 372-377*": Ibid, p.122, lines 372–377.

Chapter 13: Physiotherapy

- '"someone involved in gymnastics for those who are ill"': Though they changed it to the more modern and international *fysioterapeuterna* in 2014; www.wcpt.org/news/name-change-in-Sweden-Apr14, updated Tuesday 17 June 2014;
- 'devices you can buy and use at home': *Kegel's Exercise: Females*, Author: Physiopedia contributors, Publisher: Physiopedia, Date of last revision: 26 November 2018, 20:36. UTC, Date retrieved: 22 August 2019, 11:52 URL: www.physio-pedia.com/index.php?title=Kegel%27s_Exercise_:_Females&oldid=200899, page version ID: 200899, source: Arnold H. Kegel, MD, FACS, *Stress Incontinence and Genital Relaxation*, CIBA Clinical Symposia, Feb–Mar 1952, Vol. 4, No. 2, pp.35–5.

Chapter 15: History

- 'Dr. Elizabeth Blackwell – the first female MD to qualify from a US medical school in 1849': www.cfmedicine.nlm.nih.gov/physicians/biography_35.html;
- 'Dr. Elizabeth Blackwell … who set up the New York Infirmary for Women and Children': www.broughttolife.sciencemuseum.org.uk/broughttolife/people/elizabethgarrettanderson;
- 'The City Of London Lying-in Hospital opened for the wives of tradesmen suffering the "terrors, pains and hazards of child-birth"': www.discovery.nationalarchives.gov.uk/details/r/8786bc82-6daa-4ef5-90d2-5481d937ae7a, an account of the City of London Lying-in Hospital for Married Women, at Shaftesbury House in Aldersgate Street, Instituted 30 March 1750 v15, www.books.google.co.uk/books?id=G4xbAAAAQAAJ;
- '"It cannot but greatly move our Compassion to reflect how many unhappy Women become useless to their Families and burdensome to the Public"': Ibid;
- 'The Continence Foundation of Australia audited the socio-economic cost of incontinence': www.aihw.gov.au/reports/disability/incontinence-in-australia/contents/table-of-contents;

- 'It is also characterised by a lack of proper reporting': www.bmj.com/company/newsroom/investigation-exposes-vaginal-mesh-scandal-that-has-left-thousands-of-women-irreversibly-harmed;
- 'Eileen Baxter, who died in Edinburgh in 2016': www.scotsman.com/news-2-15012/mesh-implant-listed-as-cause-of-death-for-first-time-1-4795723;
- 'It seems strange such simple things have not always been a part of standard best practice': www.doi.org/10.1007/s00192-019-04047-z, *Development, validation and initial evaluation of patient-decision aid (SUI-PDA©) for women considering stress urinary incontinence surgery*, Hui Ling Ong, Inna Sokolova, Holly Bekarma et al., *International Urogynecology Journal*, Springer Nature, 1 January 2019 Copyright © 2019, The Author(s);
- 'the notion that black women do not feel as much pain as white women': Hoffman, K.M., Trawalter, S., Axt, J.R., Oliver, M.N., *Racial bias in pain assessment and treatment recommendations, and false beliefs about biological differences between blacks and whites*, Proc Natl Acad Sci USA, 2016;113(16):4296–4301, doi:10.1073/pnas.1516047113, also www.bbc.co.uk/news/uk-england-47115305;
- 'the grandmothers of urogynae surgery survivors ... We all owe them a great debt': www.history.com/news/the-father-of-modern-gynecology-performed-shocking-experiments-on-slaves;
- 'Samuel Pepys had a bladder stone the size of a billiard ball cut out with no anaesthetic ... in 1658': www.rmg.co.uk/discover/behind-the-scenes/blog/removing-bladder-stone-size-tennis-ball.

Chapter 17: Potty training

- 'just over one in five children wets the bed at four and a half. And just under one in 12 still do at nine and a half': Butler, R.J., Heron, J. (2008) *The prevalence of infrequent bedwetting and nocturnal enuresis in childhood: A large British cohort*, Scandinavian Journal of Urology and Nephrology 42: 257–64.

Chapter 18: Poo

- 'Faeces is a "Core Disgust Elicitor"': *Language and Food: Verbal and nonverbal experiences*, Polly E. Szatrowski, John Benjamins Publishing Company, 2014;
- 'the Peristeen anal plug is marketed as a "simple, safe and discreet aid for faecal incontinence…"': www.coloplast.co.uk/peristeen-anal-plug-en-gb.aspx#section=product-description_3, product information for Peristeen anal plug;
- 'Public poo is *unthinkable*': www.theguardian.com/uk/1999/oct/05/vivekchaudhary;
- 'bowel cancer wasn't one of the "sexy cancers", not one people spoke about': www.telegraph.co.uk/culture/tvandradio/11126835/Lynda-Bellingham-interview-Im-ready-to-let-nature-take-its-course.html;
- 'Dr Emily Rubin in Pennsylvania showed that over two-thirds (68.9 per cent) of seriously ill patients considered bowel and bladder incontinence to be grimmer (or the same) as meeting the Grim Reaper himself': Rubin, E.B., Buehler, A.E., Halpern, S.D., *States Worse Than Death Among Hospitalized Patients With Serious Illnesses*, JAMA Intern Med. 2016;176(10):1557–1559, doi:10.1001/jamainternmed.2016.4362.

Chapter 19: Stigma

- '"I like to keep my body rolled away from prying eyes, never unfold too much, tell the whole story"': Jeanette Winterson, *Written On The Body*, Vintage, 1993, p.89;
- '*Médecins Sans Frontières* states that 2 million women across the globe still live with fistula': www.msf.org.uk/issues/fistula; this page was last updated 7 April 2017;
- 'the widespread nature of incontinence … means a lack of centralised action, to call for funding or policy change': 'My bladder and bowel own my life': A collaborative workshop addressing the need for continence research, report published 2018, www.mariecurie.org.uk/globalassets/media/documents/research/publications/continence-report.pdf;

- 'Research has shown that trans patients "have an increased risk for the development of micturition disorders after sex reassignment surgery" ... and that all patients ... will need "lifelong specialized follow-up"': www.scireslit.com/Urology/AJUR-ID21.pdf cite this article: Combaz, N., Kuhn, A. *Long-Term Urogynecological Complications after Sex Reassignment Surgery in Transsexual Patients: a Retrospective Study of 44 Patients and Diagnostic Algorithm Proposal*, Am J Urol Res. 2017;2(2): 038–043;
- 'it may be difficult to get the necessary help, or hard to ask if you have not been treated fairly before by society at large, health-care professionals, or those in authority, as many transgender men and women have': www.glaad.org/reference/transgender; www.obgyn.onlinelibrary.wiley.com/10.1111/aogs.12618.

Chapter 21: Feminism

- 'FOUR HUNDRED MILLION': Global Forum on Incontinence http://www.gfiforum.com/incontinence;
- 'the International Continence Society (ICS) ... argues that the range of treatments, procedures and surgeries available means that "all patients" with stress incontinence "can be successfully treated, or, at the very least, their condition significantly ameliorated"': estimated number of people affected by incontinence, International Continence Society Fact Sheets, *A Background to Urinary and Faecal Incontinence*, www.ics.org;
- 'Diseases of inactivity are responsible for one in six deaths in the UK according to the British Heart Foundation': British Heart Foundation, Physical Inactivity and Sedentary Behaviour Report 2017, www.bhf.org.uk/-/media/files/research/heart-statistics/physical-inactivity-report---mymarathon-final.pdf.

Chapter 22: PMSL

- 'Jimmy Carr and Lucy Greeves describe humour as "the last refuge of the man in trouble"': *The Naked Jape: Uncovering the Hidden World of Jokes*, Jimmy Carr (Author), Lucy Greeves (Author), Michael Joseph; First Edition, 2 November 2006;

- '"Humour doesn't dismiss a subject, but rather, often opens that subject up for discussion"': article by Gina Barrecca www.psychologytoday.com/us/blog/snow-white-doesnt-live-here-anymore/200910/your-humor-your-strength-your-creativity-your, Your Humor = Your Strength, Your Creativity + Your Intelligence.

Chapter 23: Men

- 'women's incontinence products were still framed as a way of coping … while men were encouraged to … "take back control" of their lives': Same site, different representations of men and women: www.tena.us/on/demandware.store/Sites-Tena_US-Site/en_US/FearlessStories-Women; www.tena.us/on/demandware.store/Sites-Tena_US-Site/en_US/FearlessStories-Men.

Chapter 24: Medics

- 'That meant effectively no surgical operations involving mesh should have taken place during this period unless a particular patient's circumstances met a number of very specific conditions': www.i.emlfiles4.com/cmpdoc/9/7/2/8/1/1/files/47633_mesh-letter-to-acute-ceos-and-mds.pdf; open letter sent 09/07/2018 to Acute trust CEOs and medical directors from NHS Improvement and NHS England, Wellington House, 133–155 Waterloo Road, London.

What if you are leaky too?

- 'medical research suggests between 25 and 50 per cent of women with urinary incontinence experience sexual dysfunction': www.obgyn.onlinelibrary.wiley.com/doi/pdf/10.1576/toag.13.3.143.27665; Sinclair, A.J., Ramsay, I.N., 'The psychosocial impact of urinary incontinence in women', *The Obstetrician & Gynaecologist*, 2011;13:143–148.

Acknowledgements

To everyone at Green Tree and Bloomsbury who has read about my muff, especially my wonderful editor Charlotte Croft, who understood *PMSL* right from the start and patiently highlighted all the synonyms for fanny. Sarah Skipper and Helen Williamson for solidarity, kindness and fine edits and Jasmine Parker for all the drawings. I'm sorry I put you through it all. My agent, Julia Silk, who took me on when I was all fire and fury and helped me craft a book from it: you were right about *everything*. I hope we've created something of which we can all be proud. And my 'pen pal' Deborah Crewe – for giving good email, liking my jokes, reading an entire blog, and tricking me into writing a pitch. To be honest? I don't know what I did to deserve any of you.

My husband Robin and our boys, about whom there is too much to say and without whom it would all be worthless: you taught me what love is after all. And Mum, Dad, Alice, Rosie and Martha – sorry for all the swearing, but thank you. You taught me what love was in the first place.

The people and institutions who contributed to this book with expertise, including Elaine Miller, Mars Lord, Rachel Boyce, Katharine Lough, Nicolette Zeeman, Lois Boyle, Vicky Franks, Pippa Mundy, Patrick Campbell, Amy Peake, Mary Lynne van Poelgeest, Stephanie Taylor, Myra Robson, Kath Samson, Viv Grey, Ella Hoskin, Pelvic Roar, Freedom From Fistula, the Bladder and Bowel Community, IFCP and many people who weren't named but shared so much. The Pool (RIP) for letting me start the conversation with them. And the Naked Podcast for letting me practise baring all.

Elaine Miller, I'm so honoured that you aligned your soapbox with mine. Like everyone else in the NHS who works daily to fix leaky people, you should be showered with roses wherever you walk. #SMASHTHESTIGMA

The mighty physiotherapists, continence nurse specialists, GPs, psychologists, counsellors, midwives, surgeons, receptionists, pharmacists and other healthcare workers who have been there for me at the worst times, put me back together every which way, and offered me compassion, help and hope. Like many people you are anonymised and amalgamated here – but I hope you know that I remember you all, and will always, always be grateful for those words of encouragement (especially when the lights were about to go out). This book is for you as much as anybody else.

Mighty STBC (plus Lea) – so much more than a book group. You offered cheese, wine, and love, when I met you at my lowest ebb. And Becky Rykalski for many things, including her characteristic generosity in sharing you all with me. It *was* oh so fine.

My writing group: Ellen Hewing, Tammy Hoyle, Alex Sarll, Tamar Burman – the first to hear the grimmest bits. Thank you for not running out of my kitchen screaming.

The gorgeous souls (and great friends) who read my drafts and plans and offered insight from inside and outside their comfort zones – especially Scott Pack, Beck Bream, Catherine Baigent, John Oates, Antonia Thompson, Kath Aiken, Ellie Levenson, and Matt Shinn (despite his terrible advice on titles). Also, Kerry Smith for reading it *twice*, Jess Ruston, for friendship at 5 a.m., Rachel Harris, the nicest lady doctor of all, and Sophie Ranald, for stellar second draft advice.

And then there's the rest of you, amazing folk who were there for me at work and play, in sickness and in health, as a mum and a friend, on and off line, especially Alison, Billie, Caitlin, Cathy, Clare, Claudia, Emma, Emily, Hamira, Heidi, Leah, Mel, Neil, Sal, Sheryll, Tanya, my NCT alumni, The Kids, Mums on the Run, my colleagues, especially my millennial advisors, the boys who pre-ordered, and my personal comms team. And a shout out to Big Green Bookshop, The All Good Bookshop, and Chris Brosnahan for retweets, recommendations, and giving encouragement to a sleep-deprived customer who wanted to write *something* but couldn't work out what.

And, finally, Cath Dean: you were a fearless cheerleader. The first to read a draft and the quickest to congratulate me on it becoming an actual book. I just wish you were here to be the first to hold a copy.

Luce Brett, 02 February, 2020

Index

Page numbers in italics are illustrations.